Practical Procedures in Clinical Medicine

Practical Procedures in Clinical Medicine

Michael J. Ford

MB ChB (Hons.), MRCP (U.K.)
Senior Registrar and Honorary Clinical Tutor,
The Royal Infirmary, Edinburgh

John F. Munro

MB ChB (Hons.), FRCP (Edin.)
Consultant Physician, The Eastern General
and Edenhall Hospitals, Edinburgh
Part-time Senior Lecturer,
Edinburgh University

Foreword by
John Macleod

MB ChB, FRCP (Edin.)
Consultant Physician, Western General Hospital, Edinburgh
Consultant Physician, Royal Edinburgh Hospital
Consultant Physician, Clinic for Rheumatic Diseases, Royal Infirmary, Edinburgh

CHURCHILL LIVINGSTONE
EDINBURGH LONDON MELBOURNE AND NEW YORK 1980

CHURCHILL LIVINGSTONE
Medical Division of the Longman Group Limited

Distributed in the United States of America by
Churchill Livingstone Inc., 19 West 44th Street, New
York, N.Y. 10036, and by associated companies,
branches and representatives throughout the world.

First published 1980

ISBN 0 443 02120 1

British Library Cataloguing in Publication Data
Ford, M
    Practical procedures in clinical medicine.
    1. Diagnosis, Laboratory – Laboratory manuals
    I. Title   II. Munro, J
    616.07'5   RB37   80–40180

Printed in Great Britain by The Pitman Press, Bath

Foreword

Non-invasive investigations have burgeoned in recent years. This has re-emphasised the need for meticulous care when invasive procedures are mandatory. The latter have also increased in range and complexity in relationship not only to investigation but also to management. Every competent hospital doctor nowadays must be able to enter veins, arteries and diverse cavities and organs efficiently, with the least possible risk to the patient. It is not easy to obtain guidance about such manoeuvres. It will not be found in most comprehensive textbooks of medicine or clinical examination, and rightly so, because it would be so much more conveniently placed in a separate, readily accessible handbook. Doctors Ford and Munro have done just this by translating their extensive practical expertise into direct, concise language embellished by clear, simple drawings, to guide the clinician about the indications, execution and hazards of those practical procedures which are essential components of the practice of modern medicine.

Edinburgh, 1980   John Macleod

Preface

This book is designed to assist senior medical students, house officers and registrars in performing practical procedures safely with the minimum discomfort to their patients. It should be regarded as no more than a handbook to be read before a procedure is undertaken and, if the operator is inexperienced, should never replace close medical supervision. Indeed, it is essential that any medical students should always be supervised by a fully registered doctor while performing a potentially hazardous procedure.

Before embarking on any procedure, the necessary equipment should be checked carefully and, if assistance is required, details of the procedure explained to everyone concerned. The patient should be informed as to why the test is necessary and how it will be performed, and his full cooperation should be sought. If time and circumstances permit, it is desirable to obtain written consent from or on behalf of the patient when the procedure to be undertaken carries with it an appreciable risk.

If premedication with diazepam is required, this is best achieved orally one hour beforehand. Where deemed appropriate the laboratory staff should be informed and their help enlisted. Due deference to the importance of sterility is vital. Some procedures require only that the operator should wash his hands carefully before proceeding further. Most demand that a cap, mask and gloves be worn and that the area under attention is screened with sterile drapes.

Local anaesthesia is often required and 5 to 20 ml of 1 per cent lignocaine plain can be given with comparative safety. Always check that the local anaesthetic provided does not contain adrenaline.

Finally, following any procedure, details of the after-care and nursing observations required must be clearly explained both to the patient and the senior nurse. If problems arise, the doctor must be contacted and, if necessary, further assistance sought. Blood loss and infection are much the commonest complications and should always be borne in mind when patients fail to improve or deteriorate following invasive procedures. For this reason, the indications for any procedure should be carefully assessed in the light of the expected information or response to be gained.

Edinburgh, 1980   M.J.F.
                                                                               J.F.M.

Contents

1. Venous blood sampling

INDICATIONS

To obtain venous blood for laboratory analysis, cross-matching etc.

PRECAUTIONS

Avoid venesection through flexural eczema or areas of skin sepsis. Ensure that everything required is at hand including a tourniquet, needle, syringe, tubes, antiseptic solution and dry swabs.

Patients with coagulation disorders require special care.

The operator should wash his hands.

SITES

Antecubital fossa: the routine site

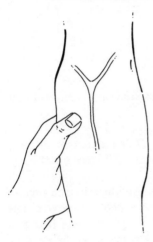

Dorsum of the hand: in difficult situations

Femoral vein: the last resort

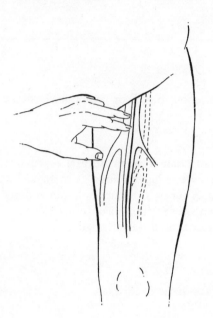

TECHNIQUE

—Apply a tourniquet well proximal to the chosen site and carefully locate the vein by palpation if necessary.

—Cleanse the skin with antiseptic solution.

—Select a suitably sized syringe and needle. When more than 20 ml of blood is required a 19 s.w.g. needle is advisable. Otherwise, a 21 s.w.g. needle is suitable.

—Insert the needle, bevel upmost, along the line of the vein at an angle of about 20° through the skin depending upon the depth of the vein. The needle enters the vein with a characteristic 'give'. Some find that during prolonged aspiration, the procedure is facilitated by bending the needle at its hilt to about 20° so that it lies in contact with the skin.

Bevel edge uppermost

—Confirm entry by aspiration of blood. If no blood is obtained, withdraw the needle very slowly while applying suction to the syringe as the needle may have transfixed the vein.

—Withdraw the required volume of blood slowly into the syringe to avoid haemolysis.

—Release the tourniquet and remove the needle after applying a dry swab over the puncture site.

—Elevate the arm with the patient applying pressure to the puncture site to minimise bruising.

—To avoid haemolysis, remove the needle before emptying the syringe into the sample tube. (If the blood was taken for blood culture, change the needle before inserting the blood into the appropriate bottles.)

SPECIAL SITUATIONS

1. Prolonged venous stasis will alter the values of the proteins, calcium, potassium and the haematocrit. In these circumstances a tourniquet is best avoided but if used, should be removed once the needle has entered the vein.

2. If it is difficult to see or palpate veins in the antecubital fossae (e.g. in the very obese) try the veins at the wrist and dorsum of the hand which may be easier to locate. If necessary, immerse the arm in warm water to facilitate venesection. If two attempts are unsuccessful, stop and ask a colleague for assistance.

The wrist is a useful alternative

3. In thin, elderly patients, immobilise the vein by skin traction proximally using the left hand. Insert the needle 1 cm distal to the proposed site of entry into the vein, preferably at a Y junction.

Immobilise the vein by traction

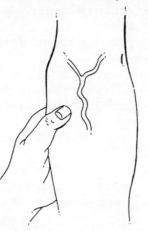

FEMORAL VEIN PUNCTURE

The femoral vein lies at the mid-inguinal point medial to the femoral artery.

Proceed to a femoral vein stab only if all else fails.

After cleansing the skin at the mid-inguinal point, insert the needle vertically just medial to the femoral artery to the depth of the needle.

Aspirate and if blood is not forthcoming, slowly withdraw the needle while applying suction.

When blood is obtained, withdraw the required amount and remove the needle, applying a dry swab to the puncture site with a firm pressure for at least three minutes.

2. Peripheral venous cannulation

INDICATIONS

Blood transfusion, hypovolaemia, septicaemia, electrolyte depletion, i.v. drug infusions.

PRECAUTIONS

Fluid overload, cardiac failure, renal failure. Before commencing check that the necessary equipment is available and that the infusion has been run through the giving set. Avoid areas of skin sepsis, eczema or burns.

The operator should wash his hands thoroughly.

TECHNIQUE

—Using a tourniquet, select a vein in the non-dominant forearm proximal to the wrist joint but avoiding the antecubital fossae where possible.

Locate a suitable vein

—If a suitable vein cannot be found, warm the limb in warm water. If necessary, the chosen vein can be made more prominent by gentle tapping or rubbing.

—Prepare the skin by shaving where necessary and cleanse with an antiseptic solution.

—In the nervous patient, inject a small bleb of 1 per cent lignocaine plain just distal to the proposed point of entry.

—Choose a suitably-sized cannula. An 18 s.w.g. needle and cannula is adequate for crystalloid solutions, e.g. N saline or 5 per cent dextrose but a 14 or 16 s.w.g. cannula is required for blood.

—Stretch the skin distally with one hand and, without touching the needle or cannula, introduce the assembly through the skin into the vein.

Insert the needle and cannula

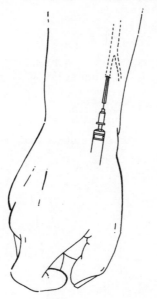

—Draw the blood back into the syringe and remove the tourniquet.

—Withdraw the needle, compressing the tip of the cannula within the vein digitally, and attach to the infusion set.

—Advance the cannula further while checking the infusion is running satisfactorily.

—Avoid contamination of the point of entry by covering the skin with a sterile dressing.

Attach the giving set

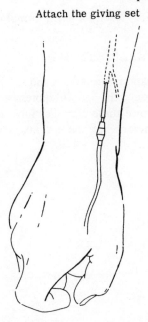

—Fix the cannula with adhesive tape avoiding the junction of the giving set and cannula since this does not prevent accidental disconnection, hampers reconnection or changes in giving set and prevents the injection of drugs into the rubber bung.

Secure with the connection exposed

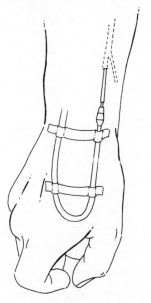

—If the cannula lies close to a joint, immobilise by splinting.

AFTER-CARE AND COMPLICATIONS

Venous inflammation, thrombosis and sepsis are common and relate to the aseptic technique, the irritant potential and the duration of the infusion. To minimise these complications, change the cannula at the earliest sign of redness or pain and never use the same vein for longer than three days.

3. Venous cut-down

INDICATIONS

When no other intravenous sites are available for the insertion of percutaneous cannulae and the operator is not experienced in central vein cannulation.

PRECAUTIONS

Before commencing, check that the necessary equipment is available. Most hospitals have pre-packed cutdown packs which include curved artery forceps, dissecting forceps, scissors, scalpel and needle holder.

SITES

Medial malleolus: the long saphenous vein lies just anterior to the medial malleolus.

The ankle

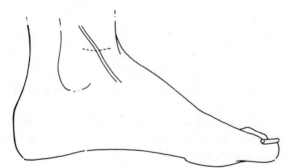

The ante-cubital fossa

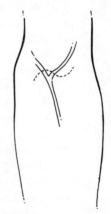

Antecubital fossa: use either the median cubital vein or the cephalic vein.

Wrist: the cephalic vein as it crosses the radio-carpal joint in the anatomical snuff box.

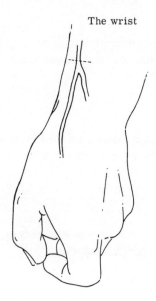

The wrist

TECHNIQUE

—Shave the area, cleanse the skin with an antiseptic solution and apply a tourniquet proximally.

—Using a strict aseptic technique (mask and gloves) infiltrate the area using 1 per cent lignocaine plain and make a 2 to 3 cm transverse incision over the expected site of the vein.

—Dissect the vein clear from surrounding tissue taking care to separate the saphenous nerve at the ankle.

—Pass a loop of 3/0 chromic catgut beneath the vein and divide it into two strands.

—Firmly tie one ligature around the vein distally. Loosely tie the other proximally and hold with forceps to provide traction and control bleeding.

—Make a small V-cut in the wall of the vein with sharp-pointed scissors.

—Introduce a 30 cm 14 or 16 s.w.g. needle and cannula through a separate skin stab just distal to the incision. Withdraw the needle and insert the cannula tip into the V-cut in the vein as the proximal ligature is relaxed.

Ligature the exposed vein

Insert the cannula through
a separate incision

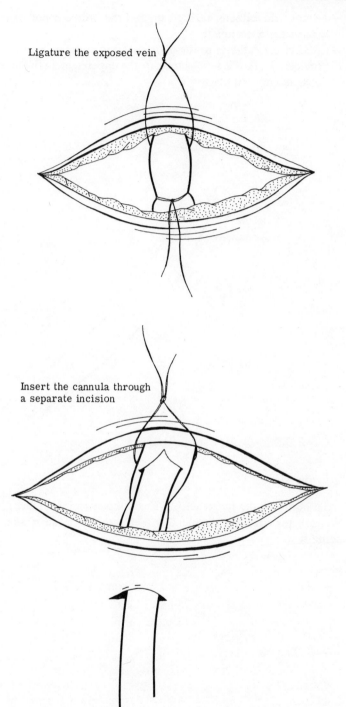

—Advance the catheter taking care that the intima is not stripped and remove the tourniquet.

—Connect the catheter to the giving set and commence infusion.

—Provided the flow is satisfactory, tie the upper ligature firmly and close the skin with 3/0 black silk.

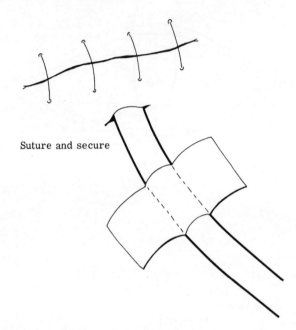

Suture and secure

—Cover the area with a sterile dressing.

COMPLICATIONS

To minimise the incidence of venous sepsis and thrombosis, remove the catheter after five days unless there are very good reasons for not doing so.

4. Arterial blood sampling

INDICATIONS

1. The assessment of acid base status in respiratory, cardiac, renal or hepatic failure.
2. Following drug overdosage or intoxication with aspirin or phenformin.
3. In assessing the presence and severity of endogenous acid overproduction, e.g. keto-acidosis, lactic acidosis.

PRECAUTIONS

Use the radial artery of the non-dominant arm because damage to the brachial or femoral arteries may result in severe limb ischaemia and the likelihood of nerve damage is remote. Prior to arterial blood sampling, inform the laboratory to minimise delay. Place the sample on ice during transit to the laboratory if delays cannot be avoided. Heparinise the syringe using $\frac{1}{2}$ ml of heparin (1000 units per ml). Expel all air bubbles from the syringe and confirm that it contains a mixer-washer. The operator should wash his hands before the procedure.

TECHNIQUE

Radial artery

—Cleanse the skin over the wrist using an antiseptic solution and inject a small bleb of 1 per cent lignocaine plain over the artery.
—While palpating the artery between the tips of the forefinger and middle finger of the left hand, introduce the needle through the skin between the fingers, at an angle of 45° and transfix the artery advancing the needle along the line of the artery. A small spurt of blood into the syringe will often be seen if a glass syringe is used but rarely using a plastic syringe.
—Withdraw 5 ml of arterial blood slowly and remove the needle.
—Press a dry swab firmly over the puncture for at least five minutes and then check to ensure that haemostasis has occurred.
—Expel any air bubbles and cap the syringe.
—Intermittently invert the syringe to ensure adequate mixing of blood and heparin.

The Radial artery

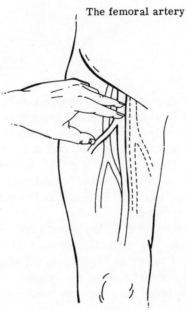

Other arteries

The technique used for the brachial or femoral artery is similar. The brachial artery lies medial to the biceps tendon and lateral to the median nerve at the apex of the ante-cubital fossa. The femoral artery lies at the mid-inguinal point medial to the femoral nerve and lateral to the femoral vein. In both sites, venous blood may be sampled and care must therefore be taken. When the brachial artery is used, extend the elbow fully over a pillow.

The femoral artery

Insert the needle vertically

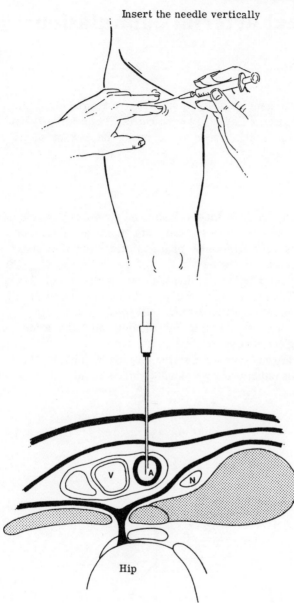

Hip

5. Peripheral arterial cannulation

In seriously ill patients who require frequent arterial blood sampling, an indwelling arterial line may be indicated. The technique should be reserved for the radial artery to minimise the risk of severe limb ischaemia.

TECHNIQUE

—Using a strict aseptic technique (mask and gloves) cleanse the skin of the wrist of the non-dominant arm with an antiseptic solution.

—Using 1 per cent lignocaine plain, infiltrate the skin and tissues surrounding the radial artery.

—Introduce a short teflon cannula with an internal needle (s.w.g. 18) obliquely through the skin and into the artery, its position being confirmed by the resulting arterial flush-back.

—Gently advance the cannula by rotation into the artery while withdrawing the needle.

—Check that arterial flow through the cannula is unimpeded.

—Compress the radial artery proximally while attaching a three-way tap.

Secure the cannula with a suture

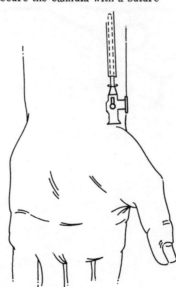

—Wash the tap and cannula through with 2 ml of Heparinised saline (5000 units per 500 ml).

—Firmly secure the cannula and tape to the skin using a 2/0 black silk ligature and cover the area with a sterile dressing.

—Thereafter when sampling, withdraw and discard the first 3 ml of blood.

—After sampling, refill the cannula with 1 ml of heparinised saline and close the tap.

Always leave the cannula heparinised

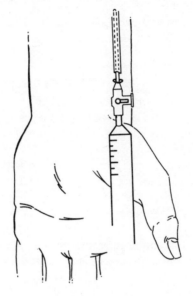

AFTER-CARE

Always leave an intra-arterial cannula exposed to ensure that accidental blood leaks will be readily detected. As soon as arterial blood samples are required only once or twice daily, remove the cannula and firmly compress the puncture site with a sterile swab for at least five minutes. Never leave the cannula *in situ* for more than five days.

6. Central venous cannulation

INDICATIONS

1. The assessment of circulatory changes in hypovolaemia, septicaemia and other causes of circulatory failure.
2. The infusion of vaso-active irritant drugs, e.g. dopamine or streptokinase.
3. The insertion of a pacing electrode or pressure transducer.
4. For parenteral nutrition.

PRECAUTIONS

—Fluid overload and cardiac failure.
—Since the use of a central venous catheter is often prolonged, cannulation through the median cubital vein at the elbow is not recommended.
—If the operator is inexperienced, expert supervision is mandatory.
—The internal jugular approach is often preferred to the subclavian route since the incidence of complications is less.
—To avoid the thoracic duct, use the right side of the neck if at all possible.
—Meticulous attention to aseptic technique is mandatory and a mask, gloves and sterile drapes should be used.

TECHNIQUE

—Place the patient supine on a bed tilted head down to distend the neck veins and avoid air-embolism.
—Turn the head away from the site at which venepuncture is planned.
—Select a suitable needle and cannula (s.w.g. 14 to 16) together with a compatible soft radio-opaque catheter 20 to 30 cm long.
—Localise the chosen vein using a 21 s.w.g. needle and syringe. Once blood is aspirated, leave the needle *in situ* and retrace the route with the larger needle and cannula.
—Never retract the cannula over the needle because of the risk of amputating the cannula tip.

The internal jugular route

The internal jugular vein lies antero-laterally in the carotid sheath and occupies a constant position between the mastoid process and the sternal end of the clavicle. It runs in a straight line deep to the sternomastoid muscle to unite with the subclavian vein to form the innominate vein.

—Cleanse the skin with an antiseptic solution and infiltrate with 1 per cent lignocaine plain at the point one-third of the distance along the line between the sternal head of the clavicle and the mastoid, just lateral to the sternomastoid muscle.

—Introduce the needle and cannula at an angle of 30 to 40° to the skin deep to the sternomastoid and advance inferiorly and medially towards the suprasternal notch until the internal jugular vein is entered at a depth of 2 to 3 cm.

—Confirm entry into the vein by aspirating blood into the syringe.

—Advance the cannula further into the vein and withdraw the needle.

—Introduce the radio-opaque catheter through the cannula to a depth of 10 to 15 cm.

—Confirm that blood can be aspirated from the catheter itself.

—Connect the catheter to the intravenous infusion and correct the head-down tilt of the bed.

—Pull the external cannula out of the skin without   moving the catheter and secure the catheter to the skin using a 2/0 black silk ligature.

—Seal the point of entry into the skin with a sterile dressing and adhesive tape.

Approaches to the deep veins

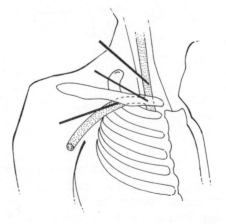

—An alternative approach to the internal jugular vein can be made from the apex of the triangle formed by the sternal and clavicular heads of sternomastoid. Direct the needle and cannula beneath the sterno-clavicular joint to pass into the vein beneath the clavicular head of sternomastoid at a depth of 2 to 3 cm.

The subclavian routes

The subclavian vein passes over the first rib behind the medial third of the clavicle to join the internal jugular vein in forming the innominate vein. The vein lies just anterior to the subclavian artery and the apical pleura.

THE INFRACLAVICULAR APPROACH

—Inject local anaesthetic 1 cm below the clavicle and just lateral to the midclavicular line.

—Introduce the needle and cannula at an angle of 15° both to the long axis of the clavicle and to the chest wall.

—Advance the needle slowly towards the sternoclavicular joint keeping close to the underside of the clavicle and above the first rib until the vein is entered at a depth of 4 to 5 cm.

THE SUPRACLAVICULAR APPROACH

—Inject the local anaesthetic into the skin at the angle between the clavicular head of sternomastoid and the clavicle.

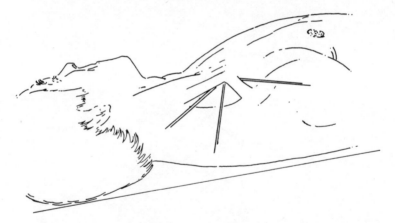

—Introduce the needle and cannula at an angle of 45° to the skin and to the clavicle at the apex of this triangle.

—Advance behind the clavicular head towards the manubriosternal joint, keeping close to the posterior aspect of the clavicle to enter the vein at a depth of 3 to 4 cm.

—Then proceed as for the internal jugular approach.

AFTER-CARE AND COMPLICATIONS

Always X-ray the chest to localise the catheter tip and exclude the presence of pneumothorax. Pneumothorax, haemothorax, air embolism, brachial plexus injuries and pericardial tamponade may occur. Remove the catheter at the first suspicion of either local or systemic infection and culture the tip of the catheter. The incidence of sepsis can be reduced by burying the catheter in a subcutaneous tunnel extending away from the entry site.

7. Central venous pressure measurement

INDICATIONS

Central venous pressure monitoring should be considered in any seriously ill patient with circulatory failure, especially if intravenous fluids are required. The central venous pressure reflects the right atrial pressure and is a useful index of right ventricular function.

PRECAUTIONS

Absolute levels of central venous pressure are of little value compared with serial changes in the c.v.p., particularly over a short period of time. Acute left ventricular failure may occur without an elevated c.v.p. A rapid rise in venous pressure following plasma expansion is potentially a sign of impending circulatory overload.

TECHNIQUE

—Following central venous cannulation, confirm radiologically that the opaque catheter tip lies satisfactorily in a great vein.
—Using a three-way tap, connect the central venous line to an infusion set and a c.v.p. manometer.

Use a fixed reference point

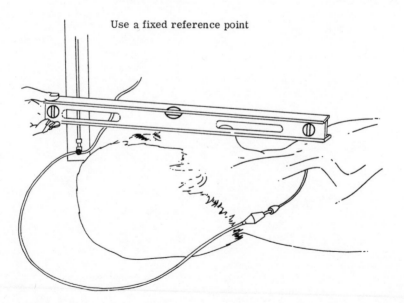

—Adjust the tap to fill the manometer and then turn the tap so that the open limb communicates with the patient.
—Observe the level at which fluid in the open limb stops falling and begins to gently rise and fall with each respiratory cycle.
—The chosen reference point is usually the manubriosternal junction but this does not reflect the absolute c.v.p. Zero the reference point on the manometer tube using a spirit level. Always re-zero this point before repeating c.v.p. recordings especially if the position of the patient has changed.

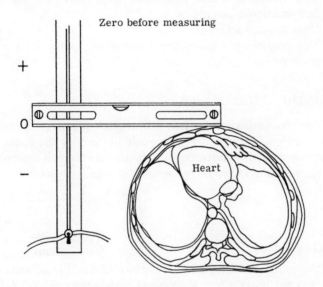

—The c.v.p. is the difference between the reference point and the level of fluid in the U-tube (either positive or negative).
—Once the c.v.p. has been measured, change the three-way tap so that the infusion continues, albeit slowly, to prevent a clot forming within the catheter. The addition of heparin 250 to 500 units to the infusion will reduce the risk of the catheter clotting or becoming infected.

8. Lumbar puncture

INDICATIONS

1. Peripheral neuropathy, especially Guillain-Barre syndrome, diabetic amyotrophy and hypertrophic polyneuropathy.
2. c.n.s. infection/neurosyphilis/meningitis (bacterial, viral or fungal).
3. Sub-arachnoid haemorrhage.
4. Disseminated sclerosis.
5. Neuroradiological procedures/lumbar myelography, air encephalography.

CONTRA-INDICATIONS

The possibility of raised intracranial pressure or spinal cord compression. Though it is important to examine the fundi, a history suggestive of raised intracranial pressure constitutes a contra-indication to the procedure even in the absence of papilloedema.

TECHNIQUE

Left lateral position

—The spinal cord terminates at the level of disc L1/L2 and the optimal entry site is in the interspace between the spines of L3/L4. This point can be identified where the line joining the highest point of the iliac crests crosses the spine.

Correct positioning is essential

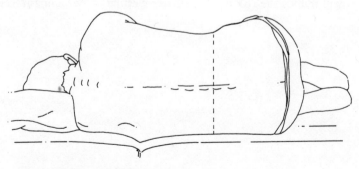

Intercrest line _ _ _ _ _

—The single most important factor is satisfactory positioning of the patient.

—Pre-medicate irritable and restless patients with i.v. diazepam.

—Arrange the patient with back flexed in the true left lateral position on the edge of the bed, supporting the right arm and right leg with pillows. (This will ensure that the position is maintained and counteract the tendency for the patient to roll over).

Use pillows to maintain
the position

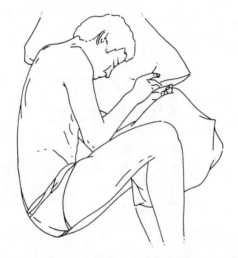

—Using the full aseptic technique (mask, gloves and sterile drapes) shave the area if necessary and cleanse with aseptic solution.

—Infiltrate the skin over the midline with 1 per cent lignocaine plain and after checking that the patient is still in the correct position, screen with sterile drapes.

—With the middle and forefingers resting on the spines of L3 and L4 respectively, introduce a 19 or 21 s.w.g. spinal needle and stylet with the bevel upmost.

—Advance the needle between the spinous processes and through the dense supraspinous ligament.

—Check to see that the needle has not been deflected and remains at 90° to the spine.

—If the line is correct, advance the needle tip through the tough ligamentum flavum to enter the subarachnoid space with a distinct 'give' at a depth of 4 to 5 cm.

—Remove the stylet and wait for c.s.f. to emerge. If this does not occur, rotate the needle. If fluid is not obtained, replace the stylet and repeat after advancing the needle no further than 0.5 cm.

The needle in situ

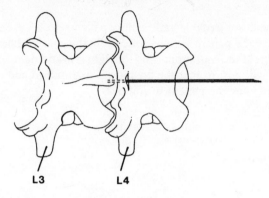

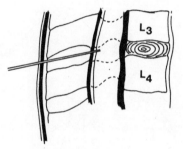

—Withdraw the needle to the skin and repeat the procedure rechecking the alignment of the needle with the spine if:
1. bony resistance is encountered
2. a nerve root is hit
3. venous blood is obtained.
—Do not have more than three attempts in any single interspace before either obtaining assistance from a senior colleague or proceeding to the L2–3 interspace.
—When c.s.f. emerges, attach the needle to the manometer by a three-way tap and with the patient relaxed, measure the pressure (normal 80 to 180 mm of c.s.f.).
—Collect the c.s.f. from the manometer together with a further aliquot to ensure that there is sufficient for the estimation of:
1. glucose (2 ml of c.s.f. in a fluoride bottle)
2. protein and electrophoresis (4 ml in a plain bottle)
3. cell count, cytology and microbiological analysis (4 ml in a sterile bottle).
—Additional c.s.f. may be required for virology or culture for tuberculosis.

Check the needle remains horizontal
during insertion

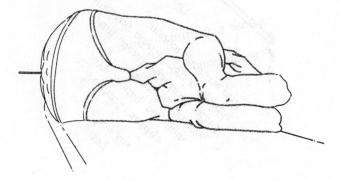

—Remove the needle and cover the puncture site with a small sterile
dressing.
—If the c.s.f. is bloodstained, centrifuge a sample to see if there is
xanthochromia.

The sitting position

The sitting position should be tried in a patient with a scoliosis or
following unsuccessful attempts in the lateral position.
—Position the patient comfortably, straddling a chair and leaning
forward to ensure that the spine is well flexed.
—Support the patient's outstretched arms with pillows.
—Proceed as above but do not measure the c.s.f. pressure in this position.

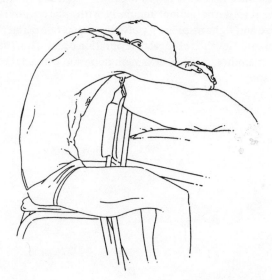

The sitting position

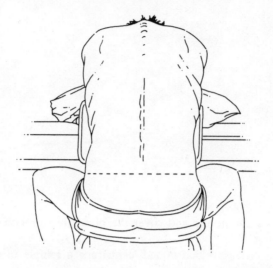

Intercrest line — — — — — —

AFTER-CARE AND COMPLICATIONS

Instruct the patient to lie prone for four hours with the foot of the bed elevated.

If headache subsequently develops, return the patient to bed for a further twelve hours.

If the c.s.f. pressure is found to be very high (i.e. greater than 250 mm of c.s.f.) review the patient regularly with quarter hourly recording of pupil size and light responses, pulse rate, respiratory rate, blood pressure and conscious level. If clinical deterioration occurs, start an infusion of 10 per cent mannitol, give i.v. dexamethasone and contact the neurosurgeons immediately.

9. Bone marrow aspiration

INDICATIONS

Any unexplained haematological abnormality which could be associated with marrow dysfunction.

PRECAUTIONS

Severe bleeding dyscrasias, e.g. haemophilia. Premedication with oral or i.v. diazepam is often useful, particularly if the sternum is the site of aspiration. A full aseptic technique must be employed using mask, gloves and sterile drapes. Sites that have been irradiated should be avoided since they will not yield marrow. Marrow aspiration from the posterior iliac crest is less hazardous and often less distressing to the patient. The risks are greater in the elderly and the osteoporotic is whom the iliac crest is the recommended site. Similarly, this site is preferable in those who may require repeated marrow aspiration, e.g. in leukaemia. However, in the obese, the posterior iliac crest may be difficult to locate and sternal aspiration is then the easier technique.

STERNAL MARROW ASPIRATION

—The site of aspiration is immediately below the manubriosternal junction, opposite the second interspace with the point of entry just to one side of the midline since a sagittal bony septum may be present.

Check the site carefully

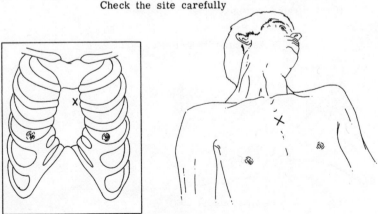

—Shave the area if necessary, cleanse with an antiseptic solution and anaesthetise the skin using 1 per cent lignocaine plain.
—Infiltrate local anaesthetic down to and including the periosteum.
—Use the anaesthetic needle to gauge the depth of the periosteum from the skin surface.
—Set the guard on the Salah needle so that it will be approximately 3 mm above the skin surface when the tip of the Salah needle touches the periosteum.

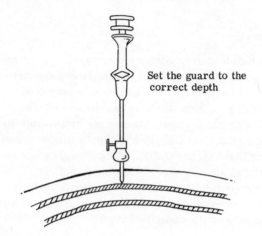

Set the guard to the
correct depth

—Using the Salah needle, draw up 2 ml of sodium citrate into a 10 ml syringe and express all but a trace to avert rapid clotting and avoid haemolysis.
—Using a firm screwing motion, penetrate the periosteum. A distinct 'give' will be felt as the needle enters the marrow cavity.
—Remove the stylet from the Salah needle and after warning the patient that they may experience chest pain, aspirate 2 ml of marrow into the 10 ml citrated syringe.

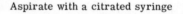

Aspirate with a citrated syringe

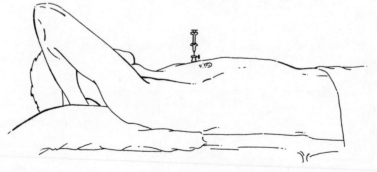

—Express this on to a watch glass and make at least eight lightly smeared marrow preparations on glass slides. (If leukaemia is suspected, remember to retain marrow blood in the appropriate preservative for chromosomal analysis).

—If the preparations appear satisfactory, remove the needle and apply firm pressure to the puncture site for three minutes.

—Cover the puncture site with a small sterile dressing.

POSTERIOR ILIAC CREST MARROW ASPIRATION

—Position the patient prone lying on a pillow placed beneath the pelvis.

Position the Patient Prone

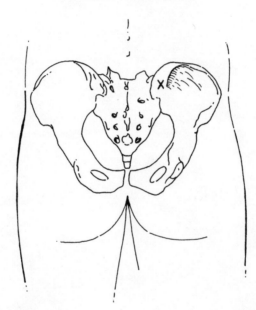

—Cleanse the skin with an antiseptic over the posterior iliac crest (often surface marked with a dimple) and screen with sterile drapes.

—Infiltrate the skin over the posterior iliac crest using 1 per cent lignocaine plain down to and including the periosteum and leave the needle *in situ*.

—Introduce the Salah needle without its guard through the skin and along the anaesthetic needle down to the periosteum.

—Remove the first needle and using a firm screwing motion, penetrate the periosteum to a depth of approximately 0.5 cm (the 'give' on entering the marrow cavity is less apparent than that using the sternal approach).

—Continue as for the sternal approach.

AFTER-CARE AND COMPLICATIONS

Complications are rare but during sternal marrow aspiration puncture of the great vessels, cardiac tamponade and pneumothorax may occur. Haematoma at the site of marrow aspiration is more likely to occur with iliac crest aspiration. Out-patients should remain in hospital for approximately one hour before being allowed home.

10. Bone trephine biopsy

INDICATIONS

1. Haematological disorders where bone marrow aspiration has been unsuccessful or marrow cytology unhelpful (e.g. myelofibrosis or malignant infiltration).
2. The diagnosis and assessment of osteomalacia and primary/secondary hyperparathyroid bone disease.

PRECAUTIONS

Severe bleeding dyscrasias. If the platelet count is less than $20 \times 10^9/l$, a platelet transfusion three hours beforehand is advisable if the bleeding time is significantly prolonged.

Premedication with oral diazepam and/or pethidine is advisable.

Avoid the iliac crest on the side on which the patient normally sleeps.

SITES

1. The anterior iliac crest.
2. The posterior iliac crest.

TECHNIQUES

A number of techniques may be used at either site. If the biopsy is indicated on haematological grounds, the posterior iliac crest is preferred

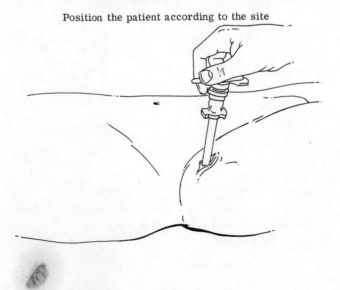

Position the patient according to the site

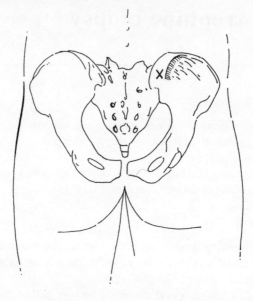

since the marrow is more cellular and either the Gardner trephine or the Jamshidi needle are suitable. When metabolic bone disease is suspected the larger Williams–Nicholson trephine may be preferable and can be used at either site.

The Williams–Nicholson trephine (5 mm diam.)

—Position the patient supine on a firm bed or couch (anterior approach).
—With full aseptic technique (mask, gloves and sterile drapes) infiltrate

The Williams - Nicholson trephine

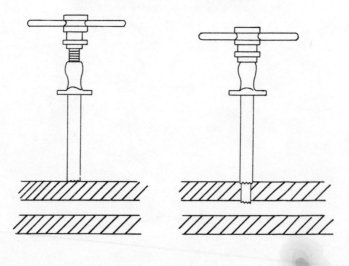

the skin over the iliac crest 3 cm posterior to the anterior superior iliac spine using 1 per cent lignocaine plain down to and including the periosteum.

—Through a 2 cm skin incision, insert further local anaesthetic into the periosteum which is then incised and deflected.

—Hold the outer toothed tube of the Williams–Nicholson trephine firmly on to the crest with the left hand and rotate the inner toothed tube clockwise into the bone with the right hand.

—Remove the trephine and biopsy by circular rocking movements and express the specimen using a stylet.

—Oversew the periosteum with chromic catgut, close the wound with 3/0 black silk and cover with a sterile dressing.

The Gardner trephine (2 mm diam.)

—Position the patient prone lying on a pillow beneath the pelvis (posterior approach).

—Under local anaesthesia, introduce the Gardner trephine and stylet through a stab incision vertically into the posterior iliac crest using a firm screwing motion.

The Gardner trephine

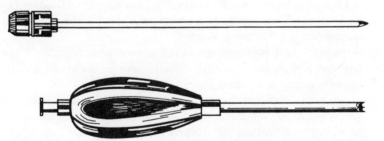

—Remove the stylet and aspirate the bone marrow if required.

—Advance the trephine fully into the bone, (3 cm) using a clockwise screwing motion.

—Remove the trephine and biopsy as for the Williams–Nicholson technique.

—The bone biopsy obtained should be sent to pathology in buffered formalin where undecalcified and decalcified sections will be prepared.

AFTER-CARE AND COMPLICATIONS

Bruising may be minimised by lying the patient on the operated side for an hour after the procedure. With regular simple analgesics, discomfort at the biopsy site rarely persists for more than two days. Remove the stitches after five days.

11. Aspiration of joints and bursae

INDICATIONS

1. The diagnosis of arthropathies especially if septic or crystal arthritis is suspected.
2. The removal of blood, pus or joint fluid.
3. The injection of corticosteroids into the joint space.
4. The injection of agents to induce a medical synovectomy.
5. The injection of contrast for arthrography.

CONTRAINDICATIONS

Severe bleeding dyscrasias, e.g. haemophilia.

GENERAL CONSIDERATIONS AND PRECAUTIONS

Strict aseptic technique is mandatory, using a mask, gloves and drapes.

Choose as large a needle as practical since synovial fluid and pus are both viscous. For small joints a 23/25 s.w.g. needle is appropriate and for large joints a 19/21 s.w.g. needle.

Though local anaesthesia is often unnecessary, infiltrate 1 per cent lignocaine plain down to and including the joint capsule if difficulties are anticipated or encountered.

Intra-articular corticosteroids are contraindicated if joint sepsis is suspected. When indicated, the doses *normally* employed are 30 to 60 mg of methylprednisolone (50–100 mg of hydrocortisone) for large joints and 10 to 30 mg of methylprednisolone (10 to 50 mg of hydrocortisone) for small joints. Since methylprednisolone can be injected in higher doses per unit volume and has a longer duration of action, it may be preferable to hydrocortisone.

Aspirate as much synovial fluid as possible.

Send samples for polarising light microscopy, protein rheumatoid factor and complement estimations and microbiological culture in plain sterile tubes and fluid for white cell counts in small sequestrenated tubes.

AFTER-CARE AND COMPLICATIONS

After the procedure, the patient should moderate his activities for the rest of the day. Haemarthrosis or joint sepsis following the procedure are extremely rare. Occasionally, an acute microcrystalline arthropathy may occur following the injection of corticosteroids.

TECHNIQUES FOR INDIVIDUAL JOINTS

Shoulder

GLENO-HUMERAL JOINT

—Aspirate using an anterior approach by introducing a 21 s.w.g. needle just below and lateral to the coracoid process through the anterior part of the deltoid.

The anterior approach

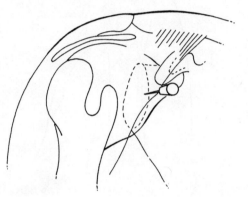

—Give injections via a posterior approach. Insert a 21 s.w.g. needle just below the lateral end of the spine of the scapula and advance medially and slightly inferiorly.

The posterior approach

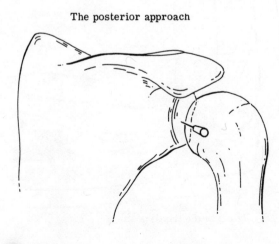

SUB-ACROMIAL BURSA

—Aspirate effusions and give injections with the arm adducted using a lateral approach through the upper part of the deltoid and below the lateral aspect of the acromion.

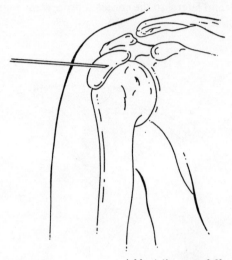

Adduct the arm fully

Elbow

HUMERO-ULNAR JOINT

—Flex the elbow to 90°, insert a 23 s.w.g. needle between the olecronon and the lateral epicondyle and advance antero-medially.

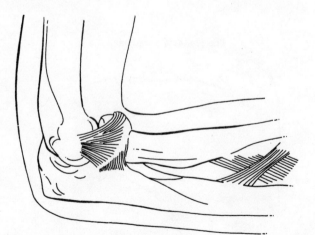

Inject in the flexed position

SUPERIOR RADIO-ULNAR JOINT

—Flex the elbow to 90° and pass a 23 s.w.g. needle into the gap between the lateral epicondyle and the head of the radius, to enter the synovial cavity which is usually continuous with that of the humero-radial and humero-ulnar joints.

MEDIAL/LATERAL EPICONDYLITIS

—Locate the tender spot at the origins of the forearm flexors or extensors by palpation.
—Inject the area with 1 per cent lignocaine plain and a corticosteroid using a 23 s.w.g. needle.

Hand

RADIO-CARPAL AND INTER-CARPAL JOINTS

—The easiest approach to the synovial cavity which is usually continuous is through the dorsal aspect of the radio-carpal joint.
—Palpate the margins of this joint and introduce the needle vertically at the distal end of the radius medial to the tendon of extensor pollicis longus.

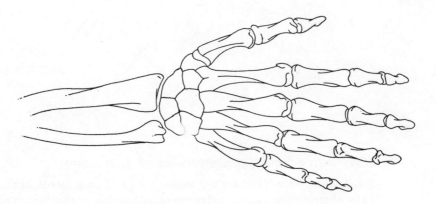

CARPAL TUNNEL SYNDROME

—Supinate the wrist and introduce a 23 s.w.g. needle at the mid point of the distal skin crease.
—Advance distally at an angle of 60° to the skin under the flexor retinaculum.

Anatomy of the carpal tunnel

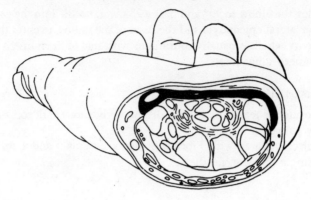

Insert needle at the mid-point
of the distal skin crease

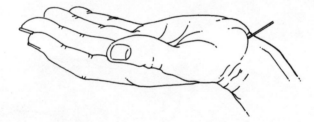

TENOSYNOVITIS OF THE TENDON OF EXTENSOR POLLICIS LONGUS

—Infiltrate the sheath but not the tendon with a 23 s.w.g. needle at the
point of tenderness just medial to the radial tubercle on the dorsum of
the wrist.

METACARPO-PHALANGEAL AND INTER-PHALANGEAL JOINTS

—With assisted gentle traction or with the joint flexed at 30°, introduce a
25 s.w.g. needle into the joint from either side of the extensor tendon.
(With the joint flexed, the joint margin lies distal to the skin crease of
the knuckle.)

Tenosynovitis of Ext. Poll. Longus

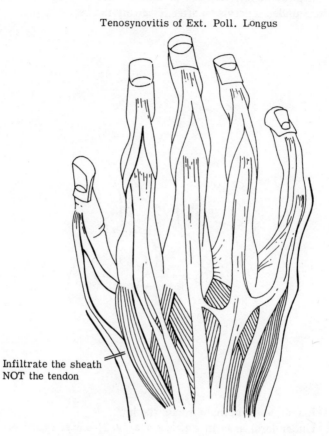

Infiltrate the sheath
NOT the tendon

Inject the flexed joint

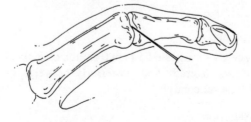

Hip joint

Aspiration/injection can be difficult and if inexperienced, should be done under supervision after reviewing the pelvic X-ray.

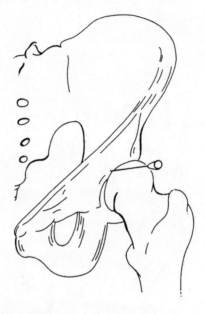

—Extend and internally rotate the hip.
—Under local anaesthesia, insert a 19/21 s.w.g. spinal needle at 60° through the skin 3 to 4 cm below the anterior superior iliac spine and 3 to 4 cm lateral to the femoral artery.
—Advance the needle posteromedially until bone is reached then withdraw slightly applying suction to the syringe.

Knee joint

KNEE EXTENDED

—Introduce a 19 s.w.g needle 1 cm from the medial border of the patella and advance laterally and posteriorly between the patella and the medial femoral condyle.

KNEE FLEXED AT 90°

—Introduce the needle medial to the patellar tendon and advance superiorly and posteriorly to enter the joint space between the femoral condyles.

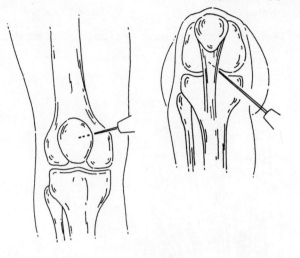

Foot

ANKLE JOINT

—Identify the joint margin with the foot plantar flexed.

—Introduce a 23 s.w.g. needle between the tendons of tibialis anterior and extensor hallucis longus in line with the joint. (Approximately 1 cm above and lateral to the tip of the medial malleolus).

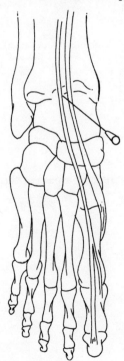

PLANTAR FASCIITIS

—Insert a 21 s.w.g. needle from either side of the heel but not through the
plantar skin.

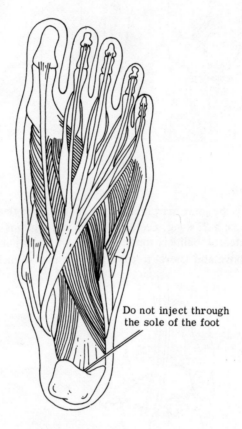

Do not inject through
the sole of the foot

—Advance the needle to the anterior aspect of the calcaneum.

12. Pleural aspiration and biopsy

INDICATIONS

1. Pleural effusion of uncertain cause.
2. Effusions causing distress.
3. Suspected empyema thoracis.

PRECAUTIONS

Severe bleeding dyscrasias, e.g. haemophilia.
Premedication is advisable and may reduce the likelihood of syncope.
Always examine the patient and check the chest X-ray before and after the procedure.

TECHNIQUE

Pleural aspiration

—Position the patient comfortably straddling a chair and slightly rotated to the opposite side to splay the ribs.

Position the patient correctly

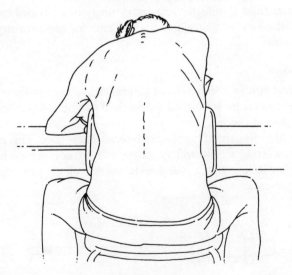

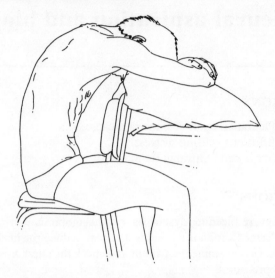

—Choose an aspiration site one intercostal space below the upper limit of
the zone of dullness to percussion in the posterior axillary line.

—Using a full aseptic technique (mask, gloves and sterile drapes) cleanse
the skin with an antiseptic solution.

—Widely infiltrate the skin and tissues down to and including the pleura
with 1 per cent lignocaine plain.

—Penetrate the pleura with the needle and aspirate to confirm the
presence of an effusion.

—If pleural biopsy is not proposed, use a 50 ml syringe, three-way tap
and 12/14 s.w.g. needle and cannula to aspirate the effusion to dryness
or until coughing or subjective distress occurs.

—Pleural fluid should be sent for cytology in a citrated container, for
microbiology in a sterile container and for biochemistry in a plain
container.

Pleural biopsy

—Pleural biopsy is indicated in pleural effusions of unknown cause but
should never be attempted unless fluid can be easily withdrawn from
the pleural space.

—The Abrams pleural biopsy needle is normally used. This comprises an
inner cutting sleeve and an outer metal trocar which has a biopsy
window in line with a round metal marker on the proximal end of the
instrument.

The Abrams needle

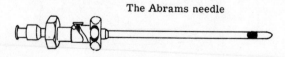

—Using a strict aseptic technique, infiltrate widely with local anaesthetic.
—Make a 1 cm scalpel incision at the aspiration site.
—Introduce the Abrams needle into the pleural space with a firm constant pressure, reducing the pressure as the distinct 'give' is felt on entering the space. (Do not rotate the trocar which has a three-sided muscle splitting point to avoid tissue damage.)
—Open the biopsy window by turning the inner sleeve fully anticlockwise.
—Using a 20 ml syringe aspirate to confirm the presence of pleural fluid and retain this fluid for laboratory analysis.
—Avoid damage to the intercostal vessels by taking biopsies *below* the horizontal.
—Withdraw the biopsy needle bringing the window of the outer trocar firmly against the inner chest wall, where it engages the parietal pleura.
—Rotate the inner trocar fully clockwise to guillotine and retain the enclosed pleural tissue.
—Remove the biopsy needle, extract the tissue and repeat the procedure to obtain two good pleural biopsies which should be sent for histological examination in buffered formalin.
—Complete the aspiration through the Abrams needle.

MALIGNANT EFFUSIONS

The rapid re-accumulation of malignant effusions may be prevented by the intra-pleural injection of 20 mg of mustine hydrochloride.

To minimise the side effects give chlorpromazine, 50 mg i.m., thirty minutes before the procedure. Aspirate the effusion as described above and then inject the mustine.

Twenty-four hours later, drain the residual effusion using an intercostal tube inserted into the most dependent part of the pleural space. This will allow the pleural surfaces to adhere firmly together and hopefully prevent a recurrence by obliterating the pleural space.

Withdraw the drain 3 to 5 days later.

COMPLICATIONS

Entry into the pleural space may produce a vasovagal syncope requiring i.v. atropine. Pneumothorax and haemopneumothorax may result. Fortunately, spontaneous resolution often follows. Rarely pulmonary oedema may complicate the rapid removal of fluid.

Always repeat the chest X-ray after the procedure and especially if the patient later becomes distressed.

13. Intercostal drainage

INDICATIONS

1. Significant pneumothorax (at least 30 per cent of hemithorax).
2. Lesser degrees of pneumothorax when associated with distress or underlying respiratory disease.
3. Recurrent or bilateral pneumothoraces.
4. Drainage of an empyema or a malignant pleural effusion.

PRECAUTIONS

Severe bleeding dyscrasia, e.g. haemophilia. Always examine the patient and the chest X-ray to confirm the presence of pneumothorax and exclude bullous emphysema. Pre-medication using oral or intravenous diazepam is recommended.

TECHNIQUE

—The optimal site for the intercostal drain is in the mid-clavicular line in the second intercostal space. In females, it may be cosmetically preferable to site the drain in the anterior axillary line in the fifth interspace.

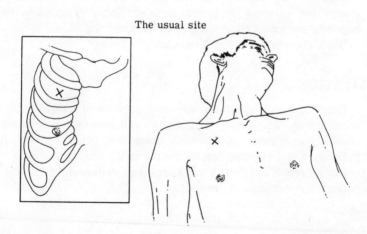

The usual site

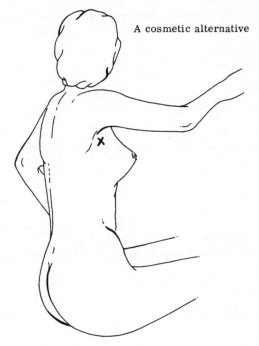

A cosmetic alternative

—For the anterior approach, seat the patient comfortably on a bed or couch.

—For the axillary approach, ask the patient to straddle a chair with the outstretched arms supported on pillows.

—Using a full aseptic technique (mask, gloves and sterile drapes) infiltrate the skin with 1 per cent lignocaine plain down to and including the parietal pleura.

—Make a 2 cm scalpel incision in the skin and underlying tissues and insert a purse-string suture around the wound using 2/0 black.

—Select a trocar and cannula which will permit the introduction of a 22 F.G. Malecot catheter.

—Introduce the trocar and cannula using firm pressure into the pleural space and then remove the trocar.

—Insert the Malecot catheter with its introducer into the pleural space.

—Remove the introducer, withdraw the cannula over the tube and pull the catheter back gently until its flange contacts the chest wall.

—Connect the drain to an underwater seal bottle (containing sterile saline to a depth of 5 cm) or to a Heimlich flutter valve.

—Wrap the ends of the purse-string suture around a swab and secure the drain using the same suture so that the ends are available to close the wound when the tube is removed.

Trocar and cannula with Malecot catheter

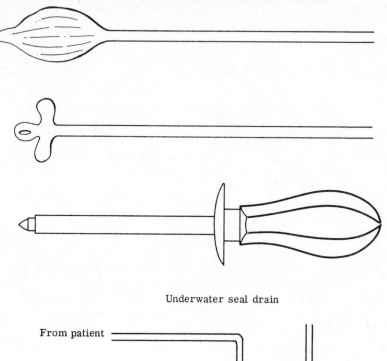

Underwater seal drain

From patient

AFTER-CARE

Confirm satisfactory positioning with a repeat X-ray.

On re-expansion the underwater seal fluid will cease to oscillate with changes in intrapleural pressure allowing the drain to be clipped off. Repeat the chest X-ray and remove the drain 48 hours after the underwater seal has ceased to oscillate provided the pneumothorax has not recurred.

Cleanse the wound with an antiseptic solution and close using the purse string suture.

Repeat the chest X-ray.

SPECIAL SITUATIONS

1. A tension pneumothorax demands urgent decompression. Use a large needle, preferably an s.w.g. 14 needle and cannula in the second intercostal space in the mid-clavicular line on the appropriate side. Then insert an intercostal drain as above.
2. In the presence of hydro- or haemo-pneumothorax, insert a lower intercostal drain to ensure complete evacuation of the intrapleural fluid.
3. If the pneumothorax is recurrent, an attempt should be made to obliterate the pleural space. This can often be achieved by injecting 10 ml of 2 per cent Camphor in oil intrapleurally before the lung is allowed to re-expand. Alternatively, talcum powder may be insufflated under a general anaesthetic. If such measures are not effective, request the help of a thoracic surgeon.
4. Failure of the pneumothorax to resolve despite a patent intercostal drain suggests the presence of either a broncho-pleural fistula or bullous emphysema without a pneumothorax. If the latter, clip off the drain and remove 48 hours later. If there is a broncho-pleural fistula, seek specialist advice.

AFTER-CARE AND COMPLICATIONS

Vaso-vagal syncope may occur requiring i.v. atropine. The patient may be pyrexial for several days. No treatment is required; indeed a local inflammatory response may aid pleurodesis.

The underwater seal bottle should never be elevated above the patient and care should always be taken that the tubes are properly connected.

Continuous suction to the drain is rarely necessary and is hazardous unless under very close supervision. Extensive subcutaneous emphysema suggests a blocked drain and requires replacement of the drain.

Trauma to intercostal vessels and rib fractures are avoidable if an appropriately sized trocar and cannula are used.

14. Bladder catheterisation

INDICATIONS

    1. Urinary retention.
    2. Monitoring urinary output in states of poor tissue perfusion.
    3. To assist the nursing care of incontinent patients with pressure sores.

PRECAUTIONS

    The risk of introducing bladder infection or inducing bacteraemia is appreciable. Patients at special risk should receive prophylactic antibiotics immediately before catheterisation. A strict aseptic technique is essential (mask and gloves).

TECHNIQUE

The urethral route

IN MALES

—Hold the penis with sterile gauze, retract the foreskin and cleanse thoroughly with an antiseptic solution using sterile swabs and dressing forceps.

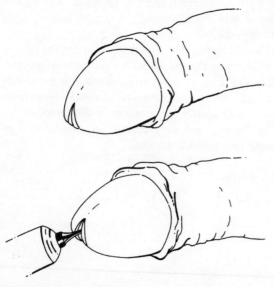

Retract the foreskin

Lubricate with anaesthetic jelly

—Insert 10 ml of 1 per cent lignocaine gel into the urethra using a sterile nozzle. Pinch the penis to prevent reflux and allow five minutes for the gel to take effect.
—Select a 14 or 16 FG Foley catheter and advance down the gel-filled urethra using forceps.

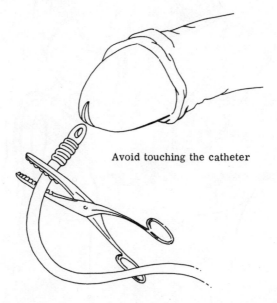

Avoid touching the catheter

—Confirm entry into the bladder and collect a urine sample for bacteriological culture and microscopy.
—Instil the volume of sterile water required to inflate the balloon as indicated on the catheter.
—Slowly drain the bladder into a urine bag.
—Always ensure that the retracted foreskin is replaced to avoid a paraphimosis.
—If difficulties are encountered move the position of the penis from the vertical to between the legs as this may facilitate its passage.
—If this fails, try a small bore Gibbon catheter (10 FG).
—If unsuccessful, do not use an introducer. Obtain assistance or proceed to a suprapubic route if indicated.

IN FEMALES

—Position the patient supine with the heels together and the knees well apart.
—Under adequate lighting, cleanse the vulva with an antiseptic solution, separating the labia with the fingers of the left hand.

Do not overfill the balloon

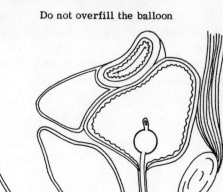

Separate and cleanse the labia

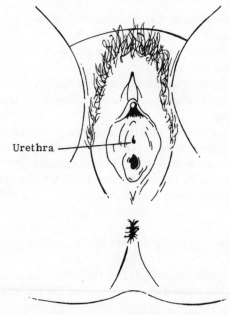

Urethra

—Hold the swab with dressing forceps, use only once and swab from anterior to posterior.

—Insert 5 ml of 1 per cent lignocaine gel into the urethra using a sterile nozzle.

—Proceed as above.

The suprapubic route

INDICATIONS

1. Urethral stricture or previous trauma.
2. Post-operative urinary diversion, e.g. bladder neck surgery.
3. In acute retention to avoid urethral damage.

CONTRAINDICATIONS

Suspected bladder carcinoma.

TECHNIQUE

—Examine the lower abdomen and proceed only when there is no doubt that the bladder is enlarged.

—Shave and cleanse the skin with antiseptic solution.

—Using full aseptic technique (mask, gloves and sterile drapes) infiltrate 1 per cent lignocaine plain into the skin 3 cm above the symphysis pubis in the midline.

—Using the same needle, enter the bladder and aspirate urine to confirm the clinical situation.

—Make a small midline stab incision 3 cm above the pubic symphysis with a scalpel.

—Use one of the commercially available cystotomy sets or a peritoneal dialysis cannula when catheterisation will only be required for several days.

—Insert the cannula and stylet through the incision and linea alba into the bladder.

—Withdraw the stylet and stitch the skin with 2/0 black silk.

—Drain the bladder into a bag and dress the wound.

—For longer periods or if bladder lavage is anticipated, use a 20/24 FG Malecot catheter.

—Select a trocar and cannula which will permit the introduction of the catheter.

—Push the trocar and cannula through the stab incision into the bladder using a firm screwing motion. (Distracting the deep tissues using artery forceps facilitates introduction.)

—Remove the trocar and insert the Malecot catheter. Then draw the cannula back over the catheter.

—Attach the catheter to a drainage tube and dress the wound. (Within weeks a tract should develop facilitating the removal and replacement of the catheter.)

Confirm bladder enlargement

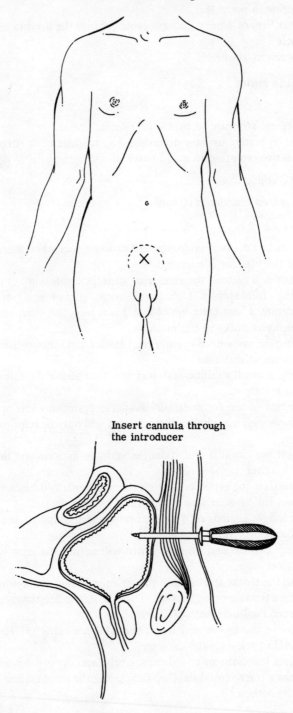

Insert cannula through
the introducer

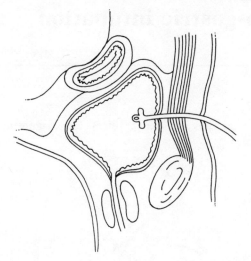

AFTER-CARE AND COMPLICATIONS

Drain the bladder slowly over several hours to reduce the risk of decompression haematuria which may occur especially with severe chronic retention.

Bladder instrumentation can produce a bacteraemia which may lead to septicaemic shock and circulatory collapse. This possibility must be considered in any patient who becomes ill following catheterisation. Blood cultures should be obtained and systemic antibiotics given if indicated.

Displacement of the suprapubic catheter may result in the extravasation of urine and perivesicular sepsis.

If a catheter is required for long-term use, regular saline bladder washouts at least twice weekly are recommended together with a change in catheter every two months.

If difficulties are encountered with urine bypassing, change the catheter every month, perform daily bladder washouts and try a spasmolytic, e.g. propantheline.

15. Naso-gastric intubation

INDICATIONS

1. The aspiration of gastric juices for diagnostic and therapeutic purposes.

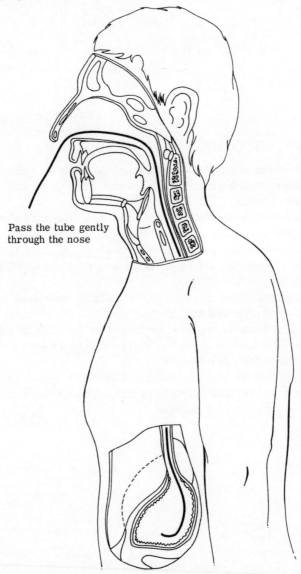

Pass the tube gently
through the nose

2. Confirmation of gastro-duodenal haemorrhage.
3. For feeding and hyperalimentation.

TECHNIQUE

—Seat the patient and inspect for nasal deformities which might impede the passage of the tube. Remove dental plates if present.

—Select a 16–20 gauge naso-gastric tube, preferably with a radio opaque tip. If prolonged hyperalimentation is required, use a fine-bore naso-gastric tube.

—Lubricate the tube and pass horizontally backwards through the nose into the naso-pharynx.

—Extend the neck slightly as the tube is advanced further and ask the patient to swallow, if necessary assisted with sips of water.

—With patience, the tube will pass into the stomach.

—Confirm its presence by syringing air down the tube while listening over the epigastrium.

—Once in position, fix the tube to the nose with adhesive tape.

—If difficulties are encountered the patient should be encouraged to try to pass the tube himself. Alternatively, try a smaller gauge tube.

—During gastric secretion tests, lie the patient in the left lateral position to facilitate the recovery of gastric juices.

AFTER-CARE AND COMPLICATIONS

Unconscious patients are at special risk of inadvertent tracheal intubation. Before gastric lavage or feeding is commenced, always check the position of the catheter tip, if necessary with an X-ray.

Regular chest physiotherapy is necessary during prolonged intubation because of the increased risk of respiratory infections; the tube should be removed as soon as is feasible.

16. Gastric lavage

INDICATIONS

1. Following acute drug overdosage.
2. In the pre-operative management of patients with pyloric stenosis.

PRECAUTIONS

The procedure is of limited value if performed beyond four hours after drug overdosage unless gastric stasis is present. The major hazard is inhalation of gastric contents. Always check that powerful suction apparatus is available and functioning beforehand.

Never perform the procedure without the prior insertion of a cuffed endotracheal tube in the unconscious patient or following ingestion of paraffin or other lipoid substances.

TECHNIQUE

Lie the patient on the left side in a three-quarter prone position on a bed or trolley in the head-down tilt and remove dental plates if present.

Position the patient in a head-down tilt

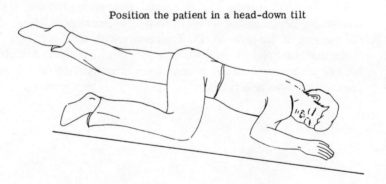

—Lubricate an 80 cm Jacques rubber tube 1 cm in diameter (size 30 English gauge).
—Pass the tube orally into the stomach with gentle but firm pressure.
—In an uncooperative patient, use dental retractors or a mouth guard to avoid the patient biting the operator's fingers or the tube itself.
—Confirm that the tube is in the stomach by auscultating over the stomach while blowing air down the tube.

—Attach a large funnel to the proximal end of the tube and siphon off the gastric contents before the lavage is commenced.

—Fill the funnel with 250 to 500 ml of luke-warm tap water and pass this into the stomach by lifting the funnel above the patient.

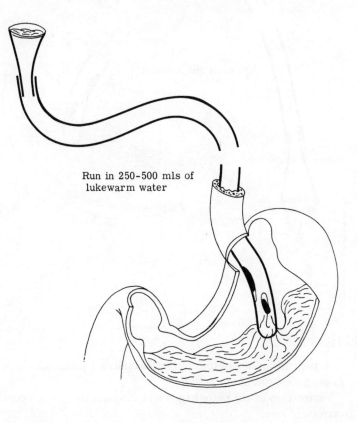

Run in 250-500 mls of lukewarm water

—Lower the funnel below the patient and siphon off the fluid into a separate bucket.

—To improve the efficiency of the lavage, gently massage the left hypochondrium to dislodge and mix tablet fragments.

—Repeat the process until the effluent is clear.

—Remove the tube taking care to occlude the tube between the fingers so that fluid within the tube will not flood into the pharynx and be aspirated.

—In the poisoned patient, examine the siphoned effluent to identify the ingested drugs and take venous blood for toxicological analysis even though this is not always used. It may prove useful in assessing the severity of poisoning, to indicate the need for specific treatment or for medico-legal purposes.

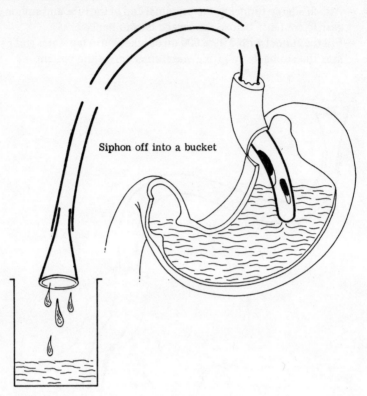

Siphon off into a bucket

COMPLICATIONS

A poor technique in uncooperative, agitated patients, will predispose to aspiration pneumonias.

Perforation of the oesophagus and stomach has been reported but is extremely rare.

Inadvertent tracheal intubation may occur in unconscious patients and reflects the failure to identify patients who require endotracheal intubation prior to lavage.

17. Use of the Sengstaken-Blakemore/ Minnesota tube

INDICATIONS

Severe upper alimentary haemorrhage from oesophageal or gastric varices unresponsive to intravenous vasopressin.

EQUIPMENT

The Sengstaken-Blakemore tube has three lumens and two inflatable balloons. One lumen communicates with the lower gastric balloon which is spherical and is used to compress the oesophago-gastric junction. The upper oesophageal balloon is cylindrical and compresses oesophageal varices. The third lumen allows gastric contents to be aspirated. The advantage of the Minnesota tube is that it has a fourth lumen which provides access to secretions collecting in the oesophagus.

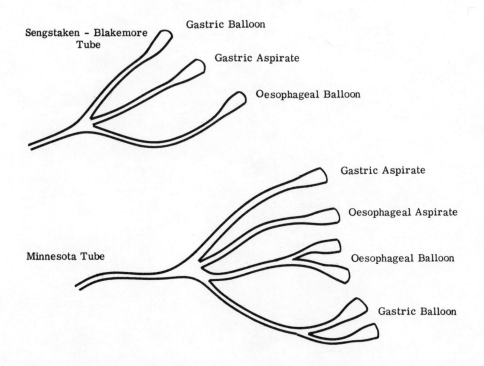

PRECAUTIONS

Before passing the tube, carefully check both balloons after inflation to ensure the absence of leaks. Label the proximal ends of the lumens clearly.

Regular pharyngeal or oesophageal aspiration and mouth toilet are necessary because oesophageal occlusion prevents the normal swallowing of saliva and exposes the patient to an inhalation hazard.

In patients with a hiatus hernia, the gastric balloon may enter the oesophagus and cause oesophageal tears or even asphyxia. Always check the position of the inflated balloons radiologically and keep a pair of scissors readily available so that if the tube becomes displaced, it may be cut to facilitate its rapid removal.

TECHNIQUE

—Anaesthetise the oropharynx using 8 to 10 puffs of a 50 per cent lignocaine spray and remove any dental plates.

—Lubricate the tube and pass through the nose or mouth. (The oral route

Confirm the position of the gastric balloon by X-ray

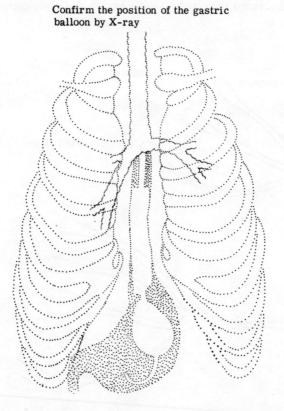

is easier but requires the use of a mouth guard to avoid the patient biting the tube.)

—Confirm that the tube has entered the stomach by injecting air down the gastric lumen.

—Fill the gastric balloon slowly with 200 to 300 ml of air, stopping if the patient develops pain.

—Check a penetrated X-ray of the lower chest/upper abdomen to confirm a satisfactory position.

—Gently withdraw the tube to pull the gastric balloon against the lower oesophageal sphincter.

—Using a sphygomomanometer, three-way tap and a 50 ml syringe, inflate the oesophageal balloon to a pressure of 30 to 40 mm of mercury then seal and leave the tap *in situ*.

—Apply 250 g of traction (half a 500 ml bag of saline) to the tube by means of a pulley attached to the head of the bed.

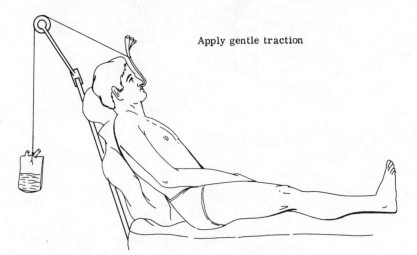

Apply gentle traction

AFTER-CARE AND COMPLICATIONS

Sedate the patient with regular i.v. diazepam as required. Aspirate the stomach and oropharynx/oesophagus hourly. Since some balloons leak slowly, check the pressure within the oesophageal balloon every hour.

To minimise the hazards of pressure necrosis, deflate the oesophageal balloon every six hours for ten minutes and then re-inflate.

If bleeding does not recur after 24 hours, deflate the oesophageal balloon and continue gastric and oesophageal aspiration hourly.

If bleeding has not occurred after 48 hours, release the tension on the tube, deflate the gastric balloon and continue hourly aspirations.

If bleeding has not occurred after 72 hours, gently remove the deflated tube.

If blood is aspirated at any stage during the three days, re-inflate both balloons and ask for surgical assistance.

Check the pressure in the oesophageal balloon regularly

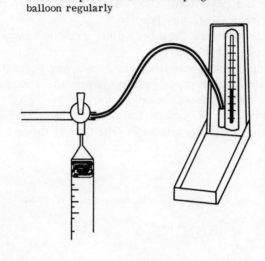

18. Peritoneal aspiration and biopsy

INDICATIONS FOR PARACENTESIS

1. The diagnosis of ascites of uncertain origin and the exclusion of bacterial peritonitis.
2. The relief of symptoms in ascites.
3. The recirculation of ascites fluid after ultrafiltration (Rhodiascit).

PRECAUTIONS

Pregnancy bleeding dyscrasias and hepatic pre-coma render the procedure hazardous. Premedication is rarely necessary and should be avoided when liver disease is suspected. Prior to the procedure, the patient should empty the bladder.

TECHNIQUES

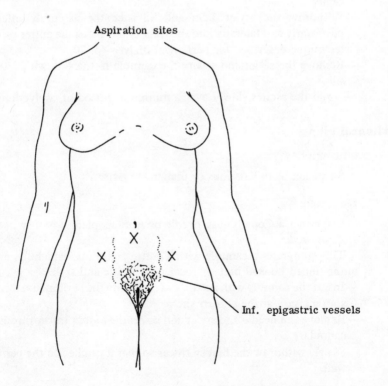

Aspiration sites

Inf. epigastric vessels

Diagnostic paracentesis

—Avoid sites of previous surgery and, to avoid the inferior epigastric vessels, use either iliac fossae at a point one-third of the distance from the anterior superior iliac spine to the umbilicus (see p. 70).

—Use a full aseptic technique (mask, gloves and sterile drapes).

—Infiltrate the overlying skin and deeper tissues down to and including the peritoneum with 1 per cent lignocaine plain.

—Using a 60 ml syringe and a 19 s.w.g. needle, aspirate fluid, if necessary by rolling the patient from the supine position towards the side of aspiration. Send the fluid for microbiological examination (sterile container), protein (and α-fetoprotein) estimation (plain tube), cell count (small sequestrenated tube) and cytological studies (citrated tube) as indicated.

Therapeutic paracentesis

—Using a full aseptic technique, infiltrate down to and including the peritoneum with local anaesthetic at a point one-third of the distance from the umbilicus to the symphysis pubis.

—Make a small transverse midline incision.

—Introduce a peritoneal dialysis cannula and stilette into the peritoneal cavity.

—Withdraw the stylet 1 cm and advance the assembly inferiorly, posteriorly and laterally into the right or left paracolic gutter using the technique described for peritoneal dialysis (p. 70).

—Remove the stylet and secure the cannula to the skin with 2/0 black silk.

—Drain the ascites slowly over a minimum period of twelve hours.

Peritoneal biopsy

INDICATIONS

Suspicion of tuberculous or malignant ascites.

TECHNIQUE

Use either a Cope biopsy needle or Abrams pleural biopsy needle.

1. Cope needle

This comprises a cannula with a cutting edge into which fits either a blunt-tipped hooked biopsy trocar or a needle and stylet.

—Insert the cannula with needle and stylet into the peritoneum through a stab incision at the chosen site.

—Remove the needle and stylet and insert the biopsy trocar through the cannula.

—Slowly withdraw the biopsy trocar so that it catches on the peritoneal wall.

Cope needle

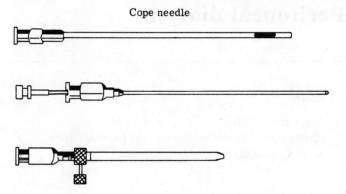

—Advance and rotate the outer cannula while firmly retracting the inner trocar to amputate the trapped peritoneum.
—Remove the biopsy trocar and place the specimen in buffered formalin.
2. *Abrams needle*
See pleural biopsy technique (p. 46).
—Insert the needle into the peritoneum through a stab incision at the chosen site.
—Open the side window of the outer trocar and oppose it against the peritoneal membrane.
—Slowly withdraw the needle along the peritoneum and rotate the inner cutting sleeve to guillotine the tissue.
—Remove the needle and place the specimen in buffered formalin.
—After draining a recurrent malignant ascites, inject 20 mg of mustine hydrochloride intraperitoneally after antiemetic sedation (e.g. chlorpromazine 50 mg i.m.).

AFTER-CARE AND COMPLICATIONS

In patients with liver disease, the rapid drainage of large volumes of ascites may precipitate hepatic encephalopathy, aggravate hypoproteinaemia and promote the rapid reaccumulation of ascites. Adequate analgesia is essential following peritoneal biopsy.

Injury to the inferior epigastric vessels, intraperitoneal bleeding and bowel or bladder perforation are rare but may require surgical intervention. Bacterial peritonitis is rare but may present de novo as recurrent hepatic ascites. Routine sampling for microbiological culture should avoid any delay in diagnosis.

19. Peritoneal dialysis

INDICATIONS

1. Acute renal failure.
2. Chronic renal failure unsuitable for haemodialysis.
3. Severe poisoning by dialysable drugs.

CONTRAINDICATIONS

Pregnancy, intra-abdominal sepsis or recent trauma, e.g. surgery.

TECHNIQUE

—Empty the bladder prior to the procedure, if necessary, by catheterisation and weigh the patient. With the patient supine, shave the lower abdomen and cleanse with an antiseptic solution.

Always ensure the bladder is empty

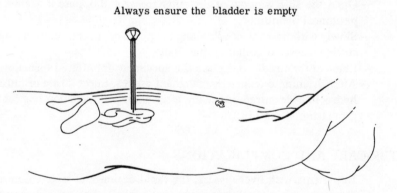

—Use a strict aseptic technique (mask, gloves and sterile drapes).
—Infiltrate the skin over the midline one-third of the distance from the umbilicus to the symphysis pubis with 1 per cent lignocaine plain down to and including the peritoneum.
—Make a small transverse stab incision and while the patient tenses the abdominal wall, insert the peritoneal cannula and stylet into the peritoneum which is entered with a characteristic 'give'.
—Withdraw the stylet 1 cm and advance the assembly inferiorly, posteriorly and laterally into the left or right paracolic gutter. If this proves difficult, infuse 1 to 2 litres of dialysis fluid into the peritoneal cavity and then proceed. If still unsuccessful, try introducing the stylet

Withdraw stylet 1cm before advancing

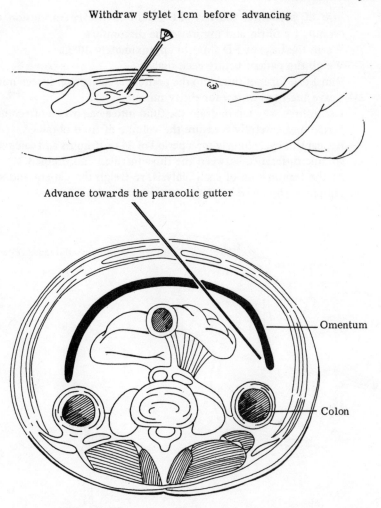

Advance towards the paracolic gutter

Omentum

Colon

and cannula in an iliac fossa one-third of the distance from the anterior superior iliac spine and the umbilicus.

—Once the assembly is correctly positioned, withdraw the stylet completely. Adjust the angle and depth of the catheter until dialysis fluid flows freely into and out of the peritoneal cavity.

—Suture the cannula to the skin using 2/0 black silk.

Dialysis procedure

—Commercially prepared peritoneal dialysis fluids are readily available. A satisfactory solution has an osmolality of 372 mmol/l with a sodium of 130 mmol/l and without added potassium.

—Add 500 units of heparin and 5 ml of 1 per cent procaine plain to each litre of peritoneal dialysis (PD) fluid to prevent occlusion of the cannula by fibrin and minimise the discomfort.

—Warm the bags of PD fluid to approximately 40°C.

—Weigh the patient before each dialysis.

—Run 1 to 2 litres of fluid into the peritoneal cavity over fifteen minutes.

—Leave the fluid *in situ* for thirty minutes.

—Use a three-way tap to drain the fluid into a bag over a fifteen minute period and carefully measure the volume of fluid obtained.

—Repeat this cycle hourly for a period of 24 to 36 hours and calculate the volume difference between the fluid instilled and drained.

—At the termination of each dialysis, re-weigh the patient and send a sample of the dialysis for microbiological culture.

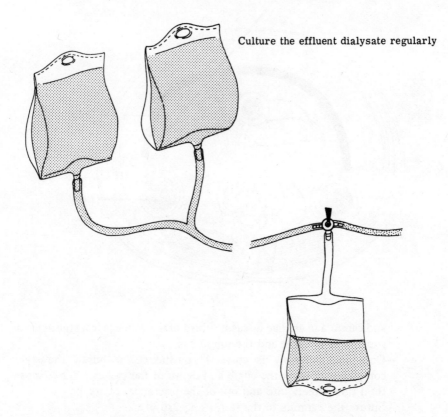

Culture the effluent dialysate regularly

FLUID AND ELECTROLYTES BALANCE

A 24 to 36 hour dialysis may result in a negative fluid balance of 2 to 3 litres or more, depending upon the number of cycles and the hypertonicity of the PD fluid. The change in the patient's weight after dialysis should provide an accurate record of fluid balance. Since the sodium concentration of the dialysate is similar to that of plasma, sodium losses can be assessed from the negative fluid balance.

With each litre of dialysate removed, 3 to 5 mmol of potassium, 100 to 200 mg of amino acid and 200 to 500 mg of protein may be lost. These losses must be taken into consideration when assessing the patient's nutritional requirements.

AFTER-CARE AND COMPLICATIONS

Perforation of bowel or bladder may occur during insertion of the PD cannula.

Abdominal discomfort during dialysis is common but may be greatly reduced by the routine addition of procaine to the PD fluid.

Bacterial peritonitis is a major complication which is usually heralded by pyrexia, abdominal pain and a cloudy dialysate and confirmed by culture of the dialysate. Its incidence can be minimised by rigid aseptic techniques during cannula manipulation, daily bacteriology of the puncture site and dialysate and by *regular changes* of cannula if peritoneal dialysis is to be continued for more than two weeks.

20. Peritoneal lavage

INDICATIONS

1. The diagnosis of intraperitoneal haemorrhage.
2. The diagnosis of acute pancreatitis with a normal serum amylase.

TECHNIQUE

—Ensure that the patient's bladder is empty; if necessary, catheterise.
—Proceed as for therapeutic paracentesis and introduce a peritoneal dialysis cannula one-third of the distance from the umbilicus to the symphysis pubis or at the lower margin of the umbilical scar.
—Withdraw the stylet and aspirate from the cannula with a 20 ml syringe. (If blood is obtained, the test is positive and lavage is unnecessary.)
—In the absence of blood, run 1 litre of warmed normal saline into the peritoneum over a ten minute period.
—Place the patient in a head-down tilt for five minutes.
—Position the patient in a feet-down tilt and siphon the fluid into a drainage bag.
—Remove the cannula and close the puncture site with a sterile dressing.

AFTER-CARE AND COMPLICATIONS

Following abdominal trauma, laparotomy is indicated if blood-stained fluid is obtained. Repeat lavage 2 to 4 hours later may be required if the emergent fluid is clear. If acute pancreatitis is suspected, send the emergent fluid for amylase estimation.

21. Small bowel biopsy

INDICATIONS

The diagnosis of gluten enteropathy and other small bowel mal-absorption states.

PRECAUTIONS

Bleeding dyscrasias: always check that the prothrombin time and platelet count are normal before proceeding.

THE CROSBY CAPSULE (WATSON MODIFICATION)

The capsule comprises a small metal cup and cap separated by a rubber diaphragm and attached to a long soft plastic catheter. The cup has a side-window and two pins, one in the side-wall and the other in the base to secure a spring-loaded cutting disc. The capsule is fired by applying suction through the attached catheter; this causes the rubber diaphragm to depress the cutting disc away from its mooring to the side-wall pin. The disc will then revolve sharply to amputate any tissue protruding through the side-window.

The Crosby capsule (Watson modification)

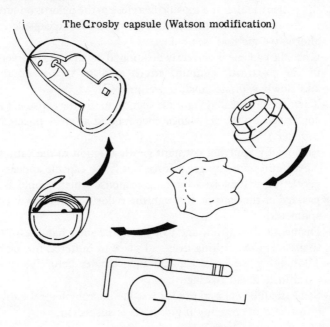

Loading the capsule

Hold the cutting disc with a metal prong and slide into the base of the cup with the cutting edge opposed to the side-wall pin so that the spring is fastened on to the base pin.

Rotate the disc anti-clockwise and withdraw slightly, thereby mooring the disc on the side-wall pin.

Cover the cup with a small rubber diaphragm (cut from a surgical glove) and gently replace the metal cap, tightening the union with a small Allen key.

TECHNIQUE

—Fast the patient overnight.

—Load the capsule, mark the catheter 100 cm from the capsule and grease with lubricant jelly.

—Ask the seated patient to swallow the capsule with the neck slightly extended and any dental plates removed. Assist with sips of water until the capsule descends into the stomach.

—Give 15 ml of metoclopamide syrup (15 mg) orally and position the patient in the right lateral on a couch.

—Tape the catheter at the 100 cm mark to the left cheek and ask the patient to swallow as much of the free loop as possible.

—Establish the position of the capsule by X-ray screening after one hour.

—If the capsule is still within the stomach, either move the catheter and the patient so that the capsule lies close to the pylorus on screening and re-X-ray after a further hour OR withdraw the capsule and use the alternative method (see below).

—Once the capsule is correctly positioned beyond the ligament of Treitz in the proximal jejunum, attach a 20 ml syringe to the catheter and slowly aspirate small bowel juices.

—Then apply repeated vigorous suction to fire the capsule. (This can be confirmed by the resistance encountered as air is injected down the catheter.)

—Remove by applying constant gentle traction to the catheter.

—Never pull with any great force but if the capsule appears to stick, a gentle tug will evoke a retching response which should facilitate the passage of the capsule through the pylorus or the lower oesophageal sphincter.

—Dismantle the capsule and using a needle and a hand-lens, remove the tissue from the cutting disc and place in buffered formalin.

—Thoroughly wash the capsule and catheter before storing in liquid paraffin to avoid rusting.

—Send small bowel aspirate for routine microbiological culture and for immediate microscopy if giardiasis is suspected.

Confirm the position of
the capsule by X-ray

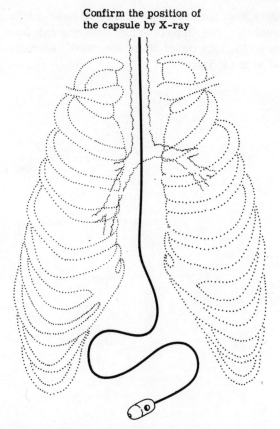

Alternative method of positioning capsule

—If difficulties in positioning the capsule are anticipated or encountered, remove the metal connector at the proximal end and pass a 16 to 18 gauge naso-duodenal tube over the catheter down to the capsule.

—Anaesthetise the pharynx using 50 per cent lignocaine spray and pass the lubricated capsule and tube through the mouth asking the patient to swallow until it lies within the stomach.

—Give 15 mg (15 ml) of metoclopamide syrup orally and after twenty minutes, establish the position of the capsule under X-ray screening.

—Gently push the tube into the correct position under screening. With patience, the pylorus can be negotiated if the capsule has not already passed into the duodenum.

AFTER-CARE AND COMPLICATIONS

Most tolerate the procedure very well and no special after-care is necessary.

Bleeding from the biopsy site and small bowel perforation are rare. Occasionally, the cup becomes disconnected from the capsule. Progress through the bowel can be monitored radiologically to facilitate retrieval from the faeces.

22. Sigmoidoscopy and rectal biopsy

INDICATIONS

1. The investigation of rectal bleeding and altered bowel habit.
2. The assessment of colitis and lower bowel neoplasm.
3. Suspected amyloidosis.

PRECAUTIONS

Avoid sigmoidoscopy during the three days preceding a barium enema because of the increased risk of bowel perforation following rectal biopsy. Satisfactory visibility of the bowel is essential during sigmoidoscopy. Never advance the instrument if vision is obscured.

Bowel preparation may alter mucosal appearances but may be necessary; it can be achieved by oral purgation on the previous evening or by the use of a disposable phospate enema one hour before the procedure.

TECHNIQUE

Position the patient comfortably

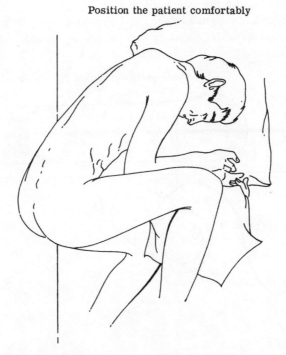

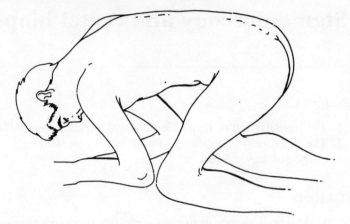

—Explain the procedure to the patient, emphasising that it may cause discomfort but should not be unduly painful.

—Position the patient on the edge of a couch in the left lateral with knees drawn up to the chest and heels well clear of the perineum. Alternatively, younger, fit patients can be examined leaning forward in the knee/elbow position.

—Examine the perianal region carefully then proceed to a digital examination of the anus and rectum to detect obvious abnormalities before passing the sigmoidoscope.

—Lubricate the sigmoidoscope and obturator and pass gently through the anal sphincter directing the instrument towards the sacrum.

The Sigmoidoscope and light-source

—Remove the obturator and attach the light source and air insufflator.

—Advance the instrument under direct vision towards the sacrum.

—Never advance unless the lumen is clearly visible and only distend the bowel with air if vision cannot otherwise be maintained.

—Identify the rectosigmoid junction, 12 to 15 cm from the anal margin where the bowel enters the pelvis at 90° to the axis of the rectum.

Change direction at the
rectosigmoid   junction

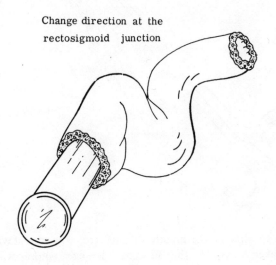

—Use the edge of the instrument to ease it past the apparent valve and advance anteriorly, to the patient's left into the sigmoid colon recording the total distance travelled from the anus.

—Throughout the procedure, carefully examine the mucosa noting its vascularity and friability as well as the presence of blood, pus, mucus and mucosal ulceration.

—Inspect any local abnormalities recording their distance from the anal margin and note the tone of the colonic wall.

—Withdraw the instrument into the lower rectum and anal canal and look for fistulae, fissures and haemorrhoids.

RECTAL BIOPSY

The peritoneum is reflected off the rectum 12 cm from the anus.

Because of the risk of intra-peritoneal perforation, never biopsy beyond 12 cm from the anal margin, use mucosal rectal biopsy forceps and always take a rectal biopsy under direct vision. When performing a rectal biopsy, lightly pinch the mucosa and pull into the lumen of the rectum. Then firmly bite, twist and retract the forceps to obtain the

Only biopsy under direct vision

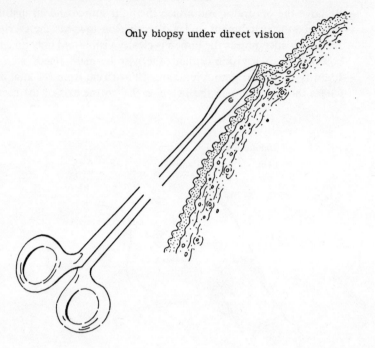

biopsy specimen recording the distance from the anus at which the biopsy was taken. Inspect the mucosal damage before withdrawing the instrument.

Place the biopsy tissue in buffered formalin for routine histology.

AFTER-CARE AND COMPLICATIONS

Perforation should not occur providing care is taken especially when the mucosa is severely inflamed.

Warn the patient to expect some degree of rectal bleeding after rectal biopsy. Profuse bleeding is rare but may require the application of a swab soaked in a weak adrenaline solution.

23. Liver biopsy

INDICATIONS

1. Investigation of hepatomegaly.
2. Assessment of liver disease and lymphoma staging.
3. Investigation of pyrexia of unknown origin.

CONTRAINDICATIONS

1. Severe bleeding dyscrasias.
2. Severe obstructive airways disease.
3. Inability to cooperate fully during the procedure.
4. Suspicion of biliary sepsis, hepatic duct obstruction, hepatic abscess, angiomatous tumour or hydatid disease.
5. When biliary tract obstruction is suspected, percutaneous trans-hepatic cholangiography under antibiotic cover is the appropriate investigation since liver biopsy is often hazardous and usually unhelpful.
6. Focal lesions involving the left lobe of the liver should only be biopsied under laparoscopic control.

PRECAUTIONS

Biopsy should not be performed by the inexperienced except under supervision.

Before biopsy, check the patient's haemoglobin, platelet count, one-stage prothrombin time and blood group and obtain blood for emergency cross-matching.

Biopsy is contraindicated if the platelet count is less than $40 \times 10^9/l$ or the prothrombin time ratio is more than 1.5.

Control any ascites as far as possible prior to liver biopsy since this can displace the liver medially and impede penetration of the liver by the biopsy needle.

If liver biopsy is necessary in biliary tract obstruction, give prophylactic antibiotics before and for five days after the procedure.

TECHNIQUE

—Premedication with oral or intravenous diazepam may be helpful.
—Use strict asepsis (mask, gloves and sterile drapes).

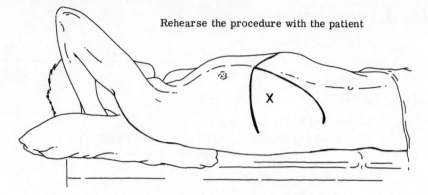

Rehearse the procedure with the patient

—Position the patient supine on the edge of the bed with the head resting on one pillow and the abducted right arm.

—Explain the procedure in detail to the patient, stressing the need to hold the breath at the end of expiration for several seconds.

—Practice this with the patient and only proceed if the patient has understood and can comply with the full instructions. ('Breathe in, breathe out, and hold your breath, hold it, hold it, all right breathe away'.)

—By percussion, localise the upper border of the liver at the end of expiration.

—Mark the biopsy site on the chest wall two intercostal spaces below this between the anterior and mid-axillary lines.

—Cleanse the right lower chest thoroughly with an antiseptic solution.

—Infiltrate the skin over the site at the upper border of the rib with 10 ml of 1 per cent lignocaine plain and then with the breath held in expiration, anaesthetise the parietal pleura, diaphragm and liver capsule.

—Make a small skin stab incision with the scalpel.

Menghini (or Jamshidi needle) technique

The Menghini needle for use in adults should be 10 cm long with a diameter of 1.6 or 1.9 mm. The proximal part of this needle contains a small obturator to prevent trauma to the specimen during aspiration. The Jamshidi needle is similar but is disposable.

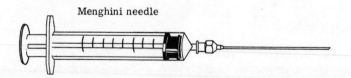

Menghini needle

—Attach the needle to a 20 ml syringe containing normal saline and express all but 2 ml of the saline.

—Advance the assembly through the skin incision down to the intercostal ligament.

—Clear any debris within the needle tip by expressing the remaining saline.

—With the patient holding the breath in full expiration, rapidly advance the needle to the depth of 8 cm from the skin surface (almost the needle's length) while simultaneously applying suction to the syringe.

'Breathe out and hold it!'
Clear the needle of debris

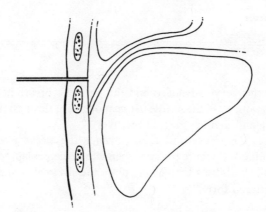

—Immediately withdraw the assembly (the entire process should take only a second to complete).

Advance while applying suction
Withdraw rapidly

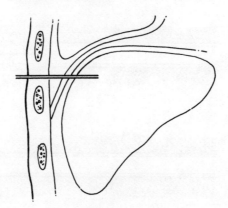

—Gently expel the sliver of tissue onto filter paper and place in buffered formalin.

—If liver tissue is required for other specific purposes, obtain a further biopsy and treat the specimen appropriately:

1. Electron microscopy – place in glutaraldehyde.
2. Immunofluorescence – place in normal saline.
3. Histochemistry – snap freeze using isopentane in liquid nitrogen.

Cutting needle biopsy (Trucut technique)

The Trucut cutting needle comprises a 10 cm pointed needle with a 2 cm notch close to its tip which is enclosed by a cutting sleeve of 2 mm diameter.

Trucut needle

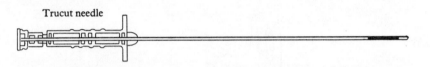

—With the sleeve advanced and the patient's breath held at the end of expiration, push the needle in one movement through the skin incision, pleura and diaphragm into the liver.

—Retract the sleeve and then advance the sleeve over the notch to guillotine and secure the specimen which has prolapsed into the notch.

—Rapidly withdraw the needle, place the sliver of tissue on filter paper in buffered formalin.

The Trucut Technique

Advance assembly

Retract sleeve

Guillotine tissue

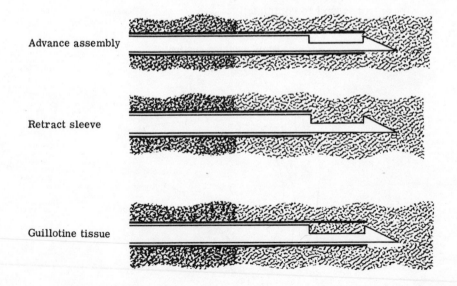

AFTER-CARE AND COMPLICATIONS

Apply a sterile dressing to the puncture site. Warn the patient that pleuritic pain may occur and to report any pain or other untoward symptoms. A dull aching discomfort in the right flank is not uncommon and may require regular simple analgesics for 24 to 36 hours.

Keep the patient supine until the following day. Record the pulse, blood pressure and respiratory rate quarter-hourly for two hours, half-hourly for two hours, hourly for four hours and then two hourly for sixteen hours.

Check a full blood count on the day following biopsy.

Pneumothorax, intraperitoneal haemorrhage, biliary peritonitis and septicaemia have all been reported following the procedure but are uncommon.

24. Renal biopsy

INDICATIONS

1. Investigation of proteinuria or suspected glomerular disease.
2. Early renal failure of uncertain origin.

CONTRAINDICATIONS

1. Inability to cooperate fully during the procedure.
2. Severe bleeding dyscrasias.
3. End-stage chronic renal failure.
4. Suspected polyarteritis nodosa because of the hazards of bleeding from renal artery aneurysms.
5. Severe hypertension.
6. In patients with only one functioning kidney.

PRECAUTIONS

The procedure requires considerable skill and should not be undertaken by the inexperienced unless under supervision.

The patient is best referred to a specialist centre to ensure that the necessary clinical expertise and laboratory facilities are available.

Before the procedure, check the patient's haemoglobin, platelet count, one-stage prothrombin time and blood group and obtain blood for emergency cross-matching.

Renal biopsy should not be performed if the platelet count is less than $40 \times 10^9/l$ or the prothrombin time ratio greater than 1.5.

TECHNIQUE

(Trucut cutting needle biopsy)
— Obtain an IVP or other radiological outline of the kidneys.
— From the radiograph, measure the distances from the centre of the lower pole of the kidney to the midline (x) and to the lower border of the twelfth rib (y) on the side to be biopsied (normally the right).
— Premedicate the patient with oral or intravenous diazepam and position prone in bed with the arms abducted and the head resting on the hands and one pillow.
— Insert a small sand-bag or rolled pillows under the abdomen so that the

Check the measurements from the X-Ray

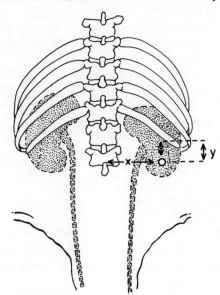

Surface-mark the biopsy site

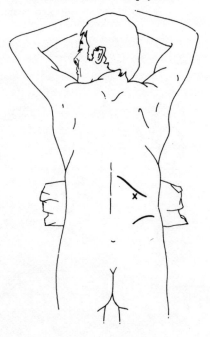

abdominal pressure holds the kidney firmly against the posterior abdominal wall.

—Using a ball pen, mark out the midline over the vertebral processes, the lower border of the twelfth rib and a line parallel to and at the measured distance x from the midline.

—Mark the biopsy site on this line at the distance y (approx. 3 cm) below the lower border of the twelfth rib depending upon the renal position.

—Using a strict aseptic technique (mask, gloves and sterile drapes) cleanse the area with antiseptic solution.

—Infiltrate 1 per cent lignocaine plain and change to a 21 s.w.g. spinal needle so that the deeper tissues, muscles and perirenal tissues can be anaesthetised.

—Advance the spinal needle while the patient is holding his breath, always ensuring that when the patient breathes, the needle is allowed to swing freely.

—Movement of the unsupported needle during respiration is confirmation that the needle tip has entered the renal substance.

—Withdraw the spinal needle noting the maximum depth of the needle tip from the skin.

—Introduce the Trucut needle vertically through a stab skin incision.

—Instruct the patient to breathe in and hold the breath.

—Advance the assembly to the depth reached by the spinal needle.

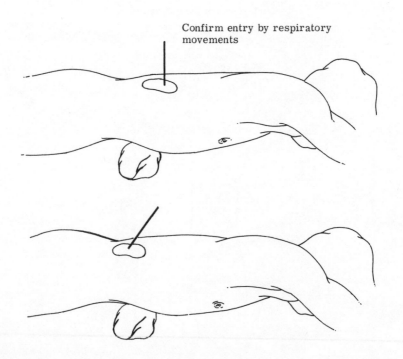

Confirm entry by respiratory movements

—Then advance the needle tip alone a further 2 cm; push the outer sleeve forward to guillotine and secure the tissue and remove the assembly. Instruct the patient to breathe normally.

—Remove the specimen carefully from the needle and cut into fragments using a scalpel.

—Renal tissue should be placed on filter paper in buffered formalin for routine histology, in glutaraldehyde for electron microscopy and in normal saline for immunofluorescent studies.

—If unsuccessful, repeat the procedure. If still unsuccessful, try again another day using an image intensifier and the screening facilities within an X-ray department.

AFTER-CARE AND COMPLICATIONS

Cleanse the skin incision with antispetic and cover with a small sterile dressing. Instruct the patient to lie prone until the following day and to drink freely to minimise the risk of clot colic.

Warn that haematuria is common and ask the patient to report any untoward symptoms.

Record the pulse, blood pressure and respiratory rate quarter-hourly for two hours, half-hourly for two hours and hourly for four hours. Check a full blood count on the following day. With experience, serious complications are uncommon but bowel perforation, retroperitoneal haemorrhage, pancreatitis and biliary peritonitis have all been reported.

25. Breast biopsy

INDICATIONS

The pre-operative confirmation of breast tumours detected on clinical examination and biplanar mammography. Its use may avoid the need for open breast biopsy.

TECHNIQUE

—Wash the hands thoroughly and then cleanse the breast with an antiseptic solution.
—Infiltrate the skin overlying the mass to be biopsied with 1 per cent lignocaine plain.
—Make a small stab incision.
—Hold the mass between the fingers of the left hand.
—Insert the Trucut cutting needle with the specimen notch covered, into the breast down to the mass.

Advance assembly down to the mass

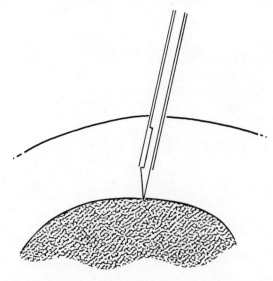

—Pass only the inner needle into the mass to a depth of 2 to 3 cm and then advance the outer cutting sleeve to guillotine and secure the breast biopsy.

Advance the inner needle into the mass

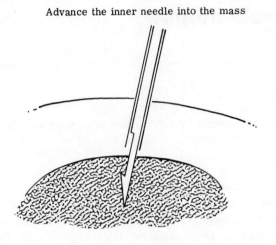

Advance the sleeve to secure the biopsy

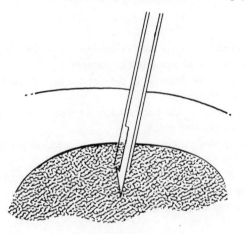

—Withdraw the assembly and compress the puncture site with a swab.
—Cover with a small sterile dressing.
—Gently remove the tissue from the needle and send for histology in buffered formalin.

AFTER-CARE

The technique is free from serious complications but local haemorrhage may occur.

26. Muscle biopsy

INDICATIONS

The identification of myopathies and neuromuscular disorders.

PRECAUTIONS

Severe bleeding dyscrasias, e.g. haemophilia. Muscle biopsy is particularly valuable in distinguishing between polymyositis and other myopathies if histochemical studies are available but is rarely justified in the absence of these facilities. Only large muscle bulks should be biopsied.

TECHNIQUE

The optimum site is vastus lateralis but the deltoid, triceps and gastrocnemius are acceptable alternatives.
—Wash the hands thoroughly then shave and cleanse the skin with an antiseptic solution.
—Infiltrate the skin and subcutaneous tissues but not the muscle with 1 per cent lignocaine plain.
—Use the Trucut cutting needle and proceed as for breast biopsy.
—Obtain two small samples for examination.
—Apply firm pressure to the biopsy site for five minutes.
—Place the sample for histochemistry in a mounting medium on a cork disc and rapidly freeze in isopentane cooled to −150°C in liquid nitrogen.
—Fix one specimen in glutaraldehyde for electron microscopy. Alternatively, place both on filter paper in a Petri dish of normal saline so that the muscle fibres may be correctly aligned using a dissecting microscope prior to fixation.

AFTER-CARE AND COMPLICATIONS

Haemorrhage and sepsis are extremely rare. The patient should be fully ambulant after muscle biopsy.

27. Respiratory resuscitation

Respiratory arrest may occur alone or in associated with cardiac arrest (see Ch. 28).

TECHNIQUES

Maintenance of airway

—Remove any dental plates and check the pharynx is clear.
—Ventilate the patient immediately either directly mouth-to-mouth or with a Brook airway.
—Position the neck in mild extension, support the jaw with one hand and pinch the nostrils with the other during chest inflation.
—Observe that the chest wall rises and falls during ventilation and aim at 12 to 15 cycles per minute.
—Check the carotid pulse regularly.
—If available, use an Ambu-bag and face mask together with a Guedel airway.
—Introduce this with the tip pointing towards the roof of the mouth for half its length and then rotate through 180° and advance fully.

Occlude the nose and support the jaw

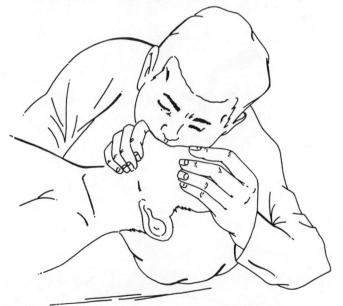

The Brook Airway

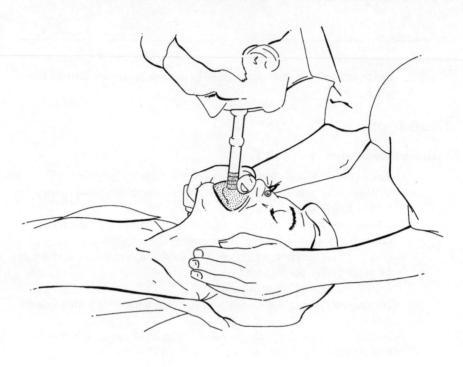

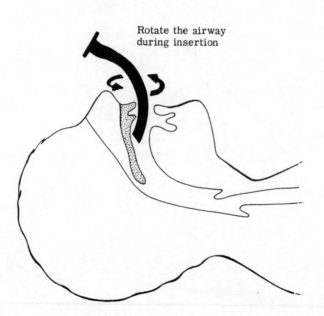

Rotate the airway
during insertion

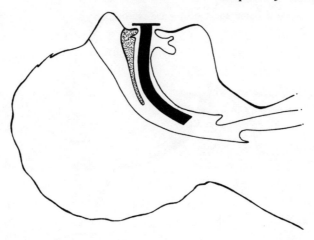

Endotracheal intubation

—Whenever possible, intubate the patient if spontaneous breathing does not return promptly.

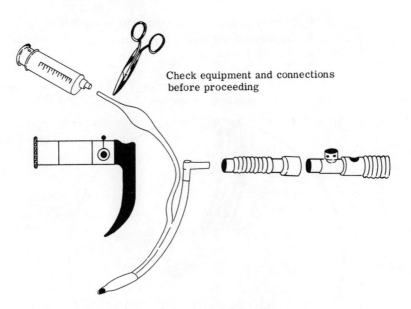

Check equipment and connections before proceeding

—Position the head on a pillow and tilt into full extension at the atlanto-occipital joint. Remove dental plates if present.

—For the right-handed operator, hold the Macintosh laryngoscope in the left hand and introduce to the right of the midline. Take care not to traumatise the teeth or lips.

Avoid damaging the lips and teeth

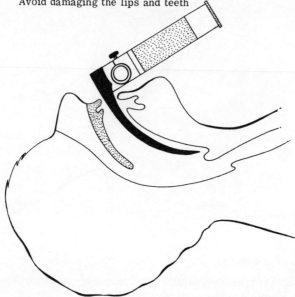

—Gently lift the tongue and jaw upwards and to the left.
—Advance the laryngoscope into the pharynx and elevate the epiglottis to reveal the larynx and vocal chords.

Elevate the epiglottis to
visualise the cords –

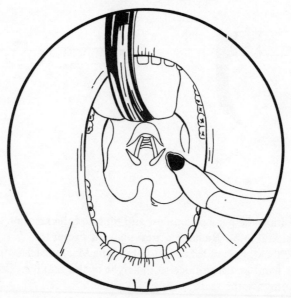

—Apply external pressure to the trachea if difficulties are encountered in visualising the vocal chords.

—Select a suitable cuffed endotracheal tube, lubricate and pass under direct vision.

—Recommended tube diameters are:

1. large adults, 9 mm
2. smaller adults and older children, 7.5 mm
3. young children, 5 mm

—Connect the endotracheal tube via a suction union adaptor, rubber tubing and metal connector to the Ambu-bag or mechanical ventilator.

—Inflate the cuff sufficiently to prevent the escape of air round the tube and clip off.

—Ensure that air entry is symmetrical on both sides of the chest by auscultation.

—Anchor the tube to the patient using a ribbon bandage and confirm that it is properly positioned radiographically.

Confirm the tube is correctly positioned

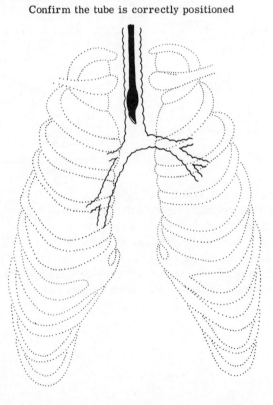

—Before removing an endotracheal tube, inspect the pharynx and aspirate any secretions.

—Deflate the cuff and as a precautionary step, insert a Guedel airway lest removal of the tube provokes a reflex contraction of the masseters.

Laryngostomy

—Laryngostomy should be performed in extreme emergencies where the upper airway is totally occluded and endotracheal intubation is not possible.

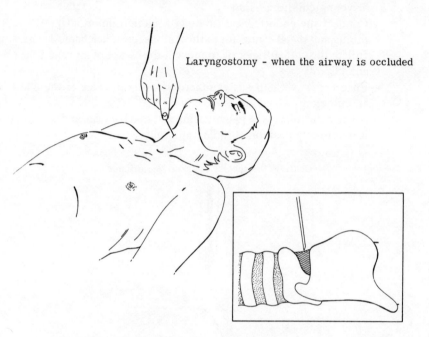

Laryngostomy - when the airway is occluded

—Use a 14 s.w.g. needle and cannula.
—Insert the assembly through the cricothyroid membrane immediately below the thyroid cartilage of the trachea.
—Remove the needle leaving the cannula *in situ*. This should allow sufficient air to pass into and out of the chest. The procedure is potentially life saving and will provide sufficient time to perform an urgent tracheostomy under general anaesthesia.

28. Cardiac resuscitation

Cardiac and respiratory arrest usually occur simultaneously but respiration may continue for some time after the heart has stopped beating. In appropriate circumstances, the absence of femoral or carotid pulses in an unconscious patient is an indication to commence external cardiac massage.

TECHNIQUE

—When a cardiac arrest occurs in hospital, alert the switchboard or a member of staff before initiating cardio-pulmonary resuscitation.
—Deliver a smart blow to the praecordium.
—Ensure that the patient is adequately supported and place a wooden board beneath the chest if necessary.

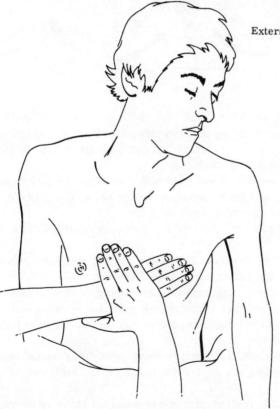

External cardiac massage

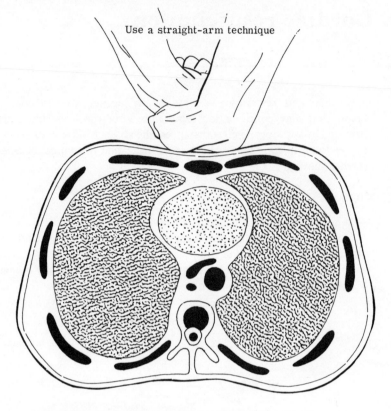

Use a straight-arm technique

—With one hand over the other, place the palm of the hand on the lower half of the sternum and depress, using a straight arm technique.

—Use the body weight to achieve cardiac massage at a rate of 60 to 80 sternal compressions per minute.

—If spontaneous respiration has ceased, ventilate the patient using a Brook airway or mouth-to-mouth respiration, applying a ratio of one ventilation to six cardiac compressions.

—When help arrives, dismiss all but two or three capable aids and screen the patient.

—Instruct one to ventilate the patient (and if possible intubate the patient) and another to prepare for defibrillation.

—Check that cardiac compression is producing a palpable pulse at the neck or groin and that a spontaneous pulse has not returned.

—Place the lubricated electrode paddles over the mid-sternum and lower left lateral chest.

—Check that no one, including yourself, is in direct contact with the patient or the bed and depress the paddles to defibrillate at 200 joules (see below).

—Obtain an e.c.g. rhythm strip and proceed thereafter as indicated.

'Stand back!'

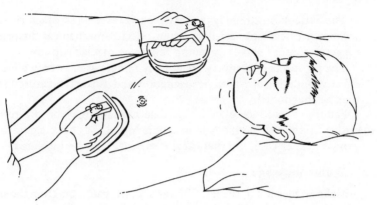

Sinus rhythm

—Administer oxygen via a polymask or MC mask.

—Set up an intravenous infusion, preferably via the external jugular vein and give 100 ml of 8.4 per cent sodium bicarbonate (100 mmol) if the arrest was prolonged.

—Check the arterial blood gases and correct any persisting acidosis with a further 50 mmol of sodium bicarbonate.

—Assume that the initial episode was ventricular fibrillation and initiate prophylactic treatment intravenously.

Supraventricular or ventricular arrhythmias

—Give the appropriate anti-arrhythmic treatment intravenously.

—Otherwise proceed as for sinus rhythm.

Continuing ventricular fibrillation

—Continue cardio-respiratory resuscitation.

—Defibrillate using 400 joules.

—Give a further 50 mmol of sodium bicarbonate and 100 mg of lignocaine as a bolus. Once the acidosis has been corrected, if necessary, defibrillate again using 400 joules.

Ventricular asystole

—Give 10 ml of 10 per cent calcium gluconate and attempt to provoke ventricular fibrillation by injecting 1 ml of 1 : 1000 adrenaline (or 1 mg of isoprenaline) either into the drip tubing or directly into the heart using a spinal needle.

—If successful, proceed as above, defibrillating with 400 joules.

SPECIAL SITUATIONS

The outlook is extremely poor if the e.c.g. reveals a satisfactory rhythm without a discernible cardiac output (electro-mechanical dissociation) suggesting either end-stage pump failure or cardiac rupture.

The prospects of recovery are equally remote after twenty minutes of effective but unsuccessful resuscitation and further measures should then be abandoned.

Failure to produce effective cardiac massage may be the result of cardiac rupture or tamponade or a non-compliant chest, e.g. asthma.

In the latter case, internal cardiac massage may be indicated.

Internal cardiac massage

—Make an incision in the left fifth intercostal space 3 cm from the sternal edge to the mid-axillary line dividing the intercostal muscles, ligament and pleura.

—Place the right hand beneath the retracted ribs and compress the heart against the sternum opening the pericardial sac if necessary.

AFTER-CARE AND COMPLICATIONS

Following successful defibrillation apply hydrocortisone cream to the paddle contact areas to reduce the local reaction which often occurs despite the use of electrode jelly.

Serious complications including cardiac tamponade are rare following successful resuscitation. A chest X-ray should be performed since cardiac failure, and rib and sternal fractures may occur especially in patients with a rigid thoracic cage.

29. D.C. cardioversion

INDICATIONS
Refractory tachyarrhythmias producing a severe reduction in cardiac output.

PRECAUTIONS
The major hazard of D.C. cardioversion is asystole. Patients previously treated with digoxin or beta-blocking drugs are especially at risk and should only be electively cardioverted where facilities for endocardial pacing are readily available.

Always try to anticipate the need for cardioversion by restricting the intravenous use of drugs in supraventricular tachycardia to those with a short plasma half-life (e.g. verapamil).

Use only 10 joules when cardioverting patients receiving digoxin and increase in 10 joules steps until successful.

If possible, perform elective cardioversion where facilities for cardiac pacing are available.

TECHNIQUE
—In the unconscious patient, undertake D.C. cardioversion without further preparation.

—In the conscious, obtain informed consent and perform under a light general anaesthetic.

—If this is not available, premedicate with 10 to 30 mg of intravenous diazepam.

—Place the patient supine and connect to an e.c.g. monitor relayed to an e.c.g.-synchronised D.C. cardioverter so that cardioversion can be triggered on the R or S wave to avoid the T wave.

—Switch on and set to deliver 50 joules for a supraventricular or 100 joules for a ventricular arrhythmia unless a lower voltage is indicated.

—Place the lubricated paddles over the mid-sternum and lower left lateral chest.

—Ensure that no one, including yourself, is in direct contact with either the patient or the bed.

—Depress the paddles to trigger the cardioversion.

—If the abnormal rhythm persists, or returns after a brief period of sinus rhythm, repeat increasing the power in 50 joules steps or less if indicated.

—Give the appropriate prophylactic treatment intravenously as soon as sinus rhythm is returned.

30. Transvenous endocardial pacing

INDICATIONS

Bradyarrhythmia associated with syncopal attacks, a low cardiac output or following myocardial infarction.

The detailed criteria for cardiac pacing are variable but include complete heart block, Mobitz type 2 second degree heart block, trifascicular block, sick-sinus syndrome and refractory supraventricular dysrhythmias.

PRECAUTIONS

Make sure all the facilites for cardio-respiratory resuscitation, external pacing and defibrillation are immediately available. Monitor the e.c.g. throughout the procedure. Give antibiotic cover to patients with suspected rheumatic or congenital heart disease before the procedure and throughout the period of pacing if an external pacemaker unit is used.

Position the bipolar pacing electrode within the heart using an image intensifier and screening facilities of an X-ray department. When these are not available, use a balloon-tipped electrode to record the intra-cardiac e.c.g. and accept the position at which a good injury pattern (ST segment elevation of at least 2 mv) and a low pacing threshold (1 v or less) are obtained.

Confirm the position of the pacing electrode with a portable chest X-ray.

TECHNIQUE

—Place the patient supine on a bed in the head-down tilt.
—Use strict asepsis (mask, gloves and sterile drapes).
—Select a suitable 30 cm cannula and check that the 90 cm bipolar pacing electrode will pass through it.
—Choose the right internal jugular or subclavian vein approach (Ch. 6). If cannulation is difficult, use the antecubital or femoral veins for rapid access.
—Infiltrate the skin with 1 per cent lignocaine plain and make a small stab incision.
—Locate the chosen vein using a 21 s.w.g. needle and syringe.
—Introduce a 16 s.w.g. intravenous infusion needle and cannula into the vein alongside the path of the first needle.
—Leave the cannula in situ but withdraw both needles.

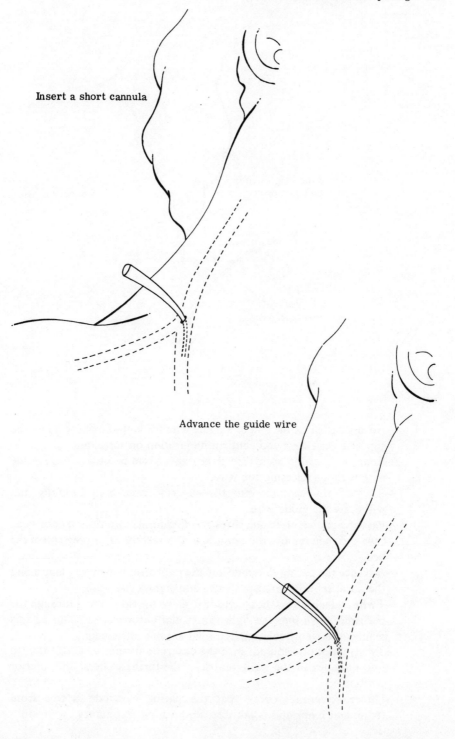

Insert a short cannula

Advance the guide wire

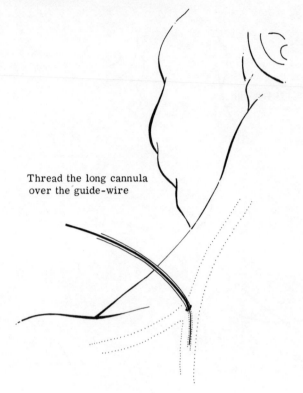

Thread the long cannula
over the guide-wire

—Advance the flexible end of a guide wire through the cannula into the
superior vena cava and confirm its position on screening.
—Remove the cannula and thread the larger 30 cm cannula over the guide
wire without releasing the wire.
—Advance the cannula into the superior vena cava carefully and
withdraw the guide wire.
—Pass the pacing electrode through the cannula into the superior vena
cava and then remove the cannula and correct the head-down tilt of the
bed.
—Advance the pacing electrode into the right atrium to make a loop along
the atrial septum, tricuspid valve and right atrial wall.
—Twist and withdraw the electrode to allow the tip to shoot through the
tricuspid valve into the right ventricular outflow tract. (During this
manoeuvre, ventricular arrhythmias are not infrequent.)
—Twist, withdraw and advance the electrode further to wedge the tip
into the apex of the right ventricle (the furthest lateral and inferior
position).
—Under screening, check that the pacing electrode is free from
redundant loops and is not displaced during respiratory excursions.

Loop the pacing electrode in the atrium

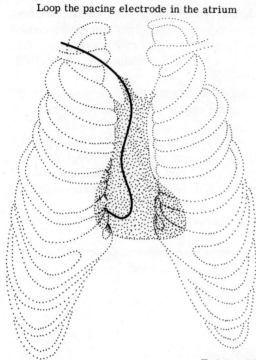

Twist, withdraw and advance the electrode

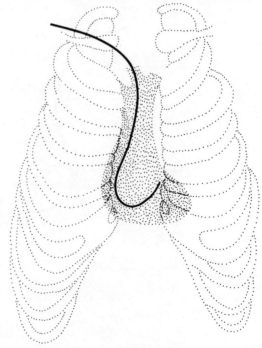

—Connect the two electrode leads to the pacing box with the sensitivity control set to detect e.c.g. voltages of 4 mv and the stimulation control to deliver 4 volts of 2 ms duration at a rate of 70 per minute. (The pacing threshold is the smallest electrical stimulus which will reliably produce ventricular capture.)

—Measure the threshold before accepting the final position of the electrode by slowly reducing the voltage from 4 volts until ventricular capture is lost.

—Reposition the electrode tip if the threshold is greater than 1 volt or if ventricular capture is lost during deep breathing or coughing.

—Once the tip is satisfactorily positioned, suture the electrode at the point of exit from the skin using 2/0 black silk taking care not to damage its insulation.

—Cleanse the area with an antiseptic solution and cover with a sterile dressing.

—Take a chest X-ray to check the electrode position and the absence of intrathoracic complications, e.g. pneumothorax.

Confirm a satisfactory position of the electrode

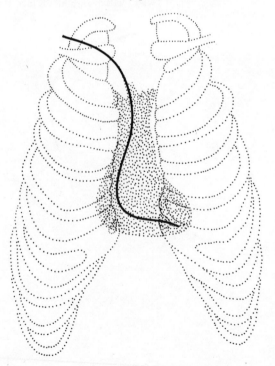

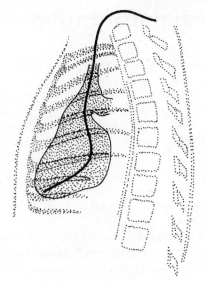

COMPLICATIONS AND AFTER-CARE

In addition to the complications of central vein catheterisation, myocardial perforation may occur and may cause retrosternal discomfort often associated with a pericardial friction rub. It is usually detected by routine chest X-ray or by loss of ventricular capture.

Ventricular tachyarrhythmias are not infrequent and may require cardioversion.

Check the pacing threshold twice daily.

A permanent internal pacemaker is indicated if cardiac pacing is required for more than ten days.

31. Pericardial aspiration

INDICATIONS

1. The rapid collection of a pericardial effusion or haemopericardium.
2. As an emergency measure in cardiac tamponade.

PRECAUTIONS

Confirm the presence of an effusion by radiology and if possible, by echocardiography.

Subtotal pericardiectomy may be necessary when effusions seem likely to recur rapidly e.g. uraemia, neoplasia and trauma.

Check that the facilities for cardio-respiratory resuscitation, including defibrillation, are immediately available before starting the procedure.

Monitor the e.c.g. throughout the pericardial aspiration.

THE ASPIRATION SITES

Anterior approach

Avoid the internal mammary arteries which run 2 cm parallel to the sternal border by aspirating in the 5th left intercostal space midway between the left sternal edge and the mid-clavicular line.

The aspiration sites

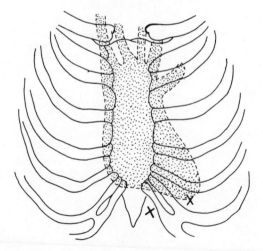

Inferior approach

Introduce the needle at 45° to the long axis of the patient between the xiphoid process and the left costal margin and direct towards the left shoulder.

The anterior approach is normally recommended since inadventent right ventricular puncture is less hazardous than left ventricular puncture. (Echocardiography may indicate the need for an inferior approach.)

TECHNIQUE

—Premedicate with intravenous diazepam.
—Use strict asepsis (mask, gloves and sterile drapes).
—Be prepared to make several attempts because fluid may be obtained from one site following a dry tap at the other.
—Position the patient sitting in bed at 45° supported by several pillows.
—Cleanse the area with an antiseptic solution and infiltrate the skin with 1 per cent lignocaine plain down to the intercostal ligament.
—Attach to 14 to 16 s.w.g. intravenous infusion needle and cannula to a 50 ml syringe and three-way tap.
—Connect the needle to the chest terminal (V) of the e.c.g. monitor using a crocodile clip.

Monitor the ECG during
the procedure

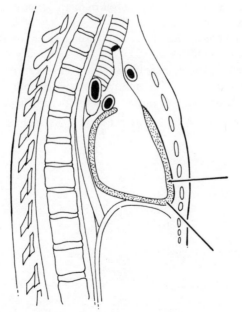

—Advance through the skin and intercostal tissues while applying suction.

—Withdraw the assembly 1 cm if heart muscle is contacted. (The e.c.g. will change to the injury pattern of marked ST segment elevation.)

—When fluid is obtained, withdraw the needle and reconnect the cannula to the three-way tap and syringe.

—Aspirate the effusion to dryness.

SPECIAL SITUATIONS

In recurrent pericardial effusions, it may help to penetrate the pericardium 10 to 15 times with the needle before aspirating to dryness to encourage the leakage of reaccumulating fluid into the mediastinum where it will be rapidly reabsorbed.

AFTER-CARE AND COMPLICATIONS

Because of the risk of pneumothorax and haemothorax, particularly associated with the anterior approach, always check the chest X-ray after the procedure.

Check the pulse rate, respiratory rate and blood pressure quarter-hourly for two hours, half-hourly for two hours and hourly for four hours thereafter.

Inadvertent right or left ventricular puncture may provoke ventricular fibrillation requiring D.C. cardioversion.

Puncture of the right atrium, pulmonary conus or coronary arteries is rare but may be life-threatening.

Rapid re-accumulation of fluid suggests a traumatic haemopericardium and indicates the need for urgent thoracotomy.

Recurrent effusions may be drained over several days if a soft, flexible cannula is left *in situ*. In this way corticosteroids and if appropriate cytotoxic drugs can be injected into the pericardial sac.

Index